Preventing Coronary Artery Disease

Cardioprotective Therapeutics in Practice

Second Edition

Preventing Coronary Artery Disease

Cardioprotective Therapeutics in Practice

Second Edition

Edited by

Martin J Kendall MD FRCP

Clinical Pharmacology Section
Department of Medicine
University of Birmingham
Queen Elizabeth Hospital
Birmingham B15 2TH, UK

Richard C Horton BSc MB FRCP

The Lancet
42 Bedford Square
London WC1B 3SL, UK

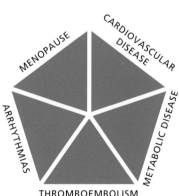

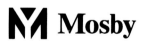 **Mosby**

St. Louis Baltimore Boston Carlsbad Chicago Naples New York Philadelphia Portland
London Madrid Mexico City Singapore Sydney Tokyo Toronto Wiesbaden

MARTIN DUNITZ

© Martin Dunitz Ltd 1994, 1998

First published in the United Kingdom in 1994 by
Martin Dunitz Ltd
The Livery House
7–9 Pratt Street
London NW1 0AE

Reprinted 1995
Second edition 1998

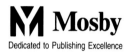

Dedicated to Publishing Excellence

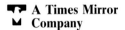

Distributed in the U.S.A. and Canada by

Mosby–Year Book
11830 Westline Industrial Drive
St. Louis, Missouri 63146

Times Mirror Professional Publishing Ltd
130 Flaska Drive
Markham, Ontario L6G 1B8

A CIP catalogue record for this book is available
from the British Library.

ISBN 1-85317-508-0

Composition by Scribe Design, Gillingham, Kent
Printed and bound in Singapore by Kyodo Printing Co (S'pore) Pte Ltd

Contents

For

Rosemary

Clarice and Ken

Contributors

Ronald Campbell BSc (Med. Sc.)Ed, MBChB FRCP
University Department of Cardiology
Freeman Hospital
Newcastle upon Tyne NE7 7DN, UK

Robert Cramb MB ChB, MSc, FRC Path
Clinical Investigation Unit
Department of Medicine
Queen Elizabeth Hospital
Birmingham B15 2TH, UK

Richard Horton BSc MB FRCP
The Lancet
42 Bedford Square
London WC1B 3SL, UK

Martin Kendall MD, MBChB, FRCP, MRCS, LRCP
Clinical Investigation Unit
Department of Medicine
Queen Elizabeth Hospital
Birmingham B15 2TH, UK

Michael Marsh MD MRCOG
University Department of Obstetrics and Gynaecology
The Royal Free Hospital
London NW3 2QG, UK

John McMurray BSc, MD, MBChB, MRCP
Department of Cardiology
Western Infirmary
Glasgow G11 6NT, UK

James Shepherd BSc, MBChB, PhD
Department of Pathological Biochemistry
Royal Infirmary
Glasgow G4 0SF, UK

Freek Verheugt MD, FACC, FESC
Academisch Ziekenhis Nijmegen
Cardiologie
6500 HB Nijmegen, The Netherlands

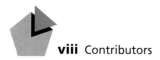

Preface

As a clinician and an editor, we are constantly struck by how few attempts are made both practically and intellectually to integrate the different therapeutic approaches to coronary artery disease into a single coherent management programme for the individual patient.

Since in most patients the first major coronary event is sudden death or a silent infarction, mortality rates can only be reduced substantially by prophylactic measures. These include lifestyle changes, with advice on smoking cessation in particular, but also, for example, on weight, diet and exercise where appropriate. Drug therapy, the subject of this book, should be offered in conjunction with and not instead of these non-pharmacological measures.

Our first aim is to argue that patients at increased risk of a coronary event and who need treatment should be offered drugs that have the potential to reduce that risk. Our emphasis has been on prophylaxis and longer term cardioprotective measures. Our second aim is to propose a broad approach to reducing coronary mortality. Patients may be at increased risk from cardiovascular disease (hypertension and angina), hyperlipidaemia and diabetes, arrhythmias, thromboembolism and, in women, the postmenopausal state. The heart can be protected from these five disorders that increase coronary risk; yet doctors, especially specialists, tend to focus on only one of these in each patient. Thus it is relatively common for patients attending a hypertension clinic not to have their plasma lipids measured or for patients attending a lipid clinic not to have hormone replacement therapy even considered as a treatment option. We believe that prevention demands an integrated approach and to emphasize this point we have coined the phrase 'a pentagon of protection'. In each chapter we have reviewed the cardioprotective evidence for each drug. We have not tried to be comprehensive but have aimed to be clinically helpful.

Martin J Kendall
Richard C Horton

Acknowledgements

A book, especially a second edition, requires the involvement of many people to bring it to successful fruition; the authors are often incidental compared with the efforts of others. We must thank Debbie Eaton for her continual and cheerful help despite the succession of rewrites and last-minute changes to the final manuscript. At Martin Dunitz Ltd, we owe a great debt to Alan Burgess and Clive Lawson. Their constant supply of good humour kept us sane at our most insecure moments and impelled us forward during times of hesitation. Finally, during our long and sometimes animated discussions about the interpretation of clinical trial data during the preparation of the first edition, Dr Rosemary Kendall provided an essential reminder that, irrespective of our often staunchly held opinions, our focus should not be deflected from the reason for this enterprise: the patient at risk from coronary heart disease.

Chapter 1
What is a cardioprotective drug?

Martin Kendall

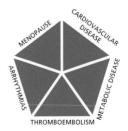

Coronary artery disease (CAD) is the most common cause of death in the developed countries of the world. It occurs more often and at an earlier age in men. Reducing the mortality and morbidity from this condition is therefore one of the most important challenges for medicine. In some developed countries, the mortality rate is falling, partly because our knowledge about risk factors is increasing and preventive measures can be taken, and partly because medical and surgical treatment of patients with known coronary disease has improved. However, the reasons for the improvement cannot be fully explained. Some developed countries still have a high coronary mortality, and some developing countries are seeing more coronary disease, though many patients with the disease remain unrecognized and untreated.

Up to half of all myocardial infarctions (MIs) are silent, being recognized only from the changes noted when serial electrocardiograms are performed on cohorts of patients who are under surveillance.[1] These patients are believed to have the same prognosis as those who have a clinically apparent infarction.[2] They are therefore at a considerable risk of recurrence, of sudden death, or of developing cardiac failure. Most of these patients are undiagnosed and are offered no treatment.

CAD is also an important cause of sudden death. In at least one in six instances, sudden death is the first, last and only manifestation of CAD.[3] The risk is greatest in hypertensives, smokers, those with left ventricular hypertrophy, and patients who have recovered from their first MI. Unless skilled help is immediately available, no form of treatment is possible.

The large numbers of patients with coronary diease who have silent infarctions or who die suddenly can only be reduced if at-risk patients are identified and preventive measures are undertaken. Efforts directed at the classic 'heart-attack' patient admitted to hospital can only assist a small proportion with coronary disease and can therefore only have a modest impact on total mortality and morbidity. To have a substantial impact, effective prophylactic measures are needed to prevent or delay the development of occlusive coronary disease and to reduce the risk of developing ventricular fibrillation.[4] Progress will only be made if our understanding of the pathological processes involved in endothelial damage, atheroma development, thrombus formation and plaque rupture translates into more effective means of limiting their effects. Lifestyle changes, particularly advice on smoking cessation, are an important part of the strategy to reduce coronary risk. There is now good evidence that non-pharmacological measures have a key role in coronary prevention. However, this book is directed specifically to the role of drugs and sets out to persuade readers to consider the preferential use of drugs that may favourably influence underlying pathology. These should be directed especially at those individuals known to be at increased risk because of, for example, hypertension or hyperlipidaemia, and those known to have coronary disease because of their past history or current symptoms.

The potential to improve the prognosis of patients known to be developing or to have CAD by appropriate drug use will only be realized if drugs with cardioprotective actions are available, if doctors are aware of the relative cardioprotective potential of the drugs they use, and if physicians are positively influenced by this property of the drug when making their choice of therapy. In practice, many doctors are unaware of the cardioprotective potential of the drugs they use and undervalue this property when selecting which agent to prescribe. The aim of this book is to overcome this obstacle to effective cardioprotective therapy.

■ THE ISCHAEMIC CYCLE

The complexity of the processes that lead to a narrowing of the coronary arteries, and ultimately to the death of patient, makes a detailed and comprehensive analysis of the possible sites for drug action impossible. However, one can describe in simple broad terms the important changes that can take place.

Risk factors for CAD combine to influence progression towards atherosclerosis and left ventricular hypertrophy. A range of ischaemic myocardial syndromes then ensues, which ultimately lead to an MI if no intervention takes place. Through several processes – neurohumoral activation, reperfusion injury and ischaemic necrosis – remodelling produces ventricular dilatation and further left ventricular dysfunction. Heart failure progresses and either an inexorable decline continues or the patient dies suddenly. Sudden death is also an important complication in the early phase after an MI.

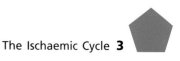

■ CARDIOPROTECTION

The use of the term 'cardioprotective drug' has fallen into disrepute, since it sounds like a marketing term that could be used without clearly defining its meaning and without providing evidence to support its use. We have used the term to denote a drug that reduces the morbidity and mortality from CAD. A patient on a cardioprotective agent should be less likely to have an MI, to reinfarct, or to die suddenly from underlying coronary disease. Drugs that reduce coronary mortality by reducing deaths from heart failure in patients with ischaemic heart disease will also be discussed, but the term cardioprotective drug will be limited to the definition given above.

To make a case that a drug is cardioprotective requires evidence, first that it has actions that would enable it to modify the processes leading to death from CAD, and second that there are adequate trial data to show that the drug has an impact on coronary mortality and morbidity in clinical practice.

Laboratory animal models have shown that stress, hypertension, free radicals and other pathological processes will lead to endothelial damage that may be a precursor for atheroma formation. Animals on atherogenic diets have been used to study atheroma formation, plaque rupture and thrombosis. A cardioprotective drug would be expected to have some positive beneficial effect on one or more of these pathological processes (Table 1.1).

The interpretation of clinical trial data has developed into a major component of epidemiology and an extremely important contributor to advances in therapeutics. This subject provokes a great deal of controversy over statistical methods, data analysis, the selection of trials to be published, and bias in the inclusion of trials for meta-analysis. Although we do not propose to enter this minefield, we will draw some practical conclusions that may assist readers.

In the Western world, pathological studies and clinical evidence suggest that CAD begins in early adult life or even earlier. Those who smoke, have positive family histories, a high blood pressure or hyperlipidaemia have more severe atheroma that involves an increasing proportion of the coronary circulation, and which gradually narrows one or more vessels. When a critical narrowing develops, the patient has an MI. If they recover, the disease progresses until an occlusion at another site occurs and the patient reinfarcts or dies. This pattern of events suggests

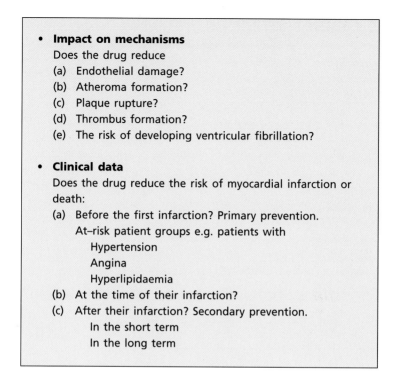

- **Impact on mechanisms**
  Does the drug reduce
  (a) Endothelial damage?
  (b) Atheroma formation?
  (c) Plaque rupture?
  (d) Thrombus formation?
  (e) The risk of developing ventricular fibrillation?

- **Clinical data**
  Does the drug reduce the risk of myocardial infarction or death:
  (a) Before the first infarction? Primary prevention.
      At–risk patient groups e.g. patients with
        Hypertension
        Angina
        Hyperlipidaemia
  (b) At the time of their infarction?
  (c) After their infarction? Secondary prevention.
      In the short term
      In the long term

Table 1.1 Evidence that a drug is cardioprotective.

that CAD is a continuous process, and it is reasonable to believe that any intervention which prevents the second infarction ought really to reduce the risk of having a first.

The second important observation is that because coronary disease is multifactorial and takes many years to develop, the modification of one contributing factor for a short time may not have an easily demonstrable impact. This would be especially true if the abnormality in question was mild and the patient population was at low risk. Thus, to demonstrate a therapeutic effect by reducing the blood pressure of mildly hypertensive, middle-aged females would be extremely difficult, and would require such large numbers of patients as to be practically impossible in a single clinical trial.

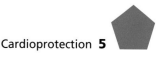

The third difficulty is that, as indicated above, many first infarctions present as sudden death or as a silent infarction. Unless all the patient population are accounted for and unless all have an ECG at the beginning and the end, the database could be very inadequate.

Secondary prevention trials are easier to perform, since a well-defined at-risk population with a relatively high mortality and morbidity is being studied. At the very least, data from these trials strongly support the case for or against a primary prevention role for a particular form of treatment. Failure to show benefit in primary prevention trials may be because the trial was too small, the treatment period was too short, the patient population was at low risk or the follow-up data were incomplete.

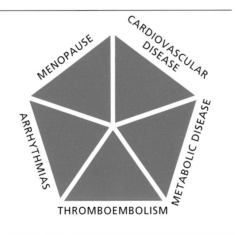

Figure 1.1 The pentagon of protection.

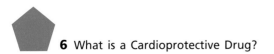

6 What is a Cardioprotective Drug?

■ THE PENTAGON OF PROTECTION

We have not written this book with the intention of producing a random collection of pharmacological facts that should be applied on an ad hoc basis to the patient with ischaemic heart disease.

We see cardioprotective therapeutics as the integrated pharmacological approach to long-term management of the patient with CAD. Thus, we have introduced the notion of a pentagon of protection around the heart. That is, we have identified five therapeutic management areas for which treatment with a cardioprotective agent would seem desirable (Figure 1.1). The five potentially treatable disorders are:

- cardiovascular disease – hypertension and angina
- metabolic disorders – particularly hyperlipidaemia and diabetes mellitus
- thromboembolism
- arrhythmias
- menopause

Methods of preventing, ameliorating or treating the effects of these processes may be seen to form a protective ring – the pentagon of protection – around the at-risk heart. Each patient should be given an individually tailored management strategy based on this concept – i.e. each side of the pentagon should be investigated and assessed to determine its contribution to the overall ischaemic risk and a strategy for intervention must be planned for each factor. The pentagon reinforces the idea that these important influences are not mutually exclusive; they are interdependent, with intervention in one area likely to affect the imperative for intervening in another; for example, hormone replacement therapy may ameliorate a lipid profile to such a degree that specific lipid-lowering treatment is not required. The pentagon can be easily incorporated into the follow-up notes of patients with CAD and serves as a reminder of the goals of treatment.

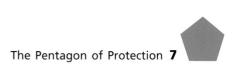

References

1. Wikstrand J, Warnold I, Toumilehto J et al, Metoprolol versus thiazide diuretics in hypertension. Morbidity results from the MAPHY study, *Hypertension* (1991) **17**:579–88.

2. Kannel WB, Abbott RD, Incidence and prognosis of unrecognised infarction: an update on the Framingham study, *N Engl J Med* (1984) **311**:1144–7.

3. Kannel WB, Cupples LA, D'Agostino RB et al, Hypertension, antihypertensive treatment and sudden coronary death: the Framingham study, *Hypertension* (1988) **II**(Suppl II):45–50.

4. Skinner JE, Regulation of cardiac vulnerability by the cerebral defence system, *J Am Coll Cardiol* (1985) **5**:88B–94B.

Chapter 2
Cardiovascular disease, hypertension and angina

Martin Kendall and John McMurray

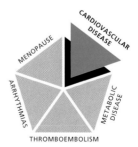

■ CARDIOVASCULAR DISEASE

Most patients with hypertension are developing coronary artery disease (CAD), patients with angina already have CAD and the majority of adults with heart failure have CAD as the cause of their disability. The management of these disorders therefore have at least two components. Thus hypertensives need to have their blood pressure controlled, angina patients need pain control and those with heart failure need symptomatic treatment to relieve their dyspnoea and oedema. The second component is the same for each group. It is to delay the progress and if possible to cause regression of their CAD and to reduce the risk of sudden death. In this chapter a number of the commonly used groups of drugs used to treat cardiovascular disorders are reviewed with the specific aim of determining and describing their capacity to reduce the mortality from CAD.

■ THIAZIDE DIURETICS

Thiazide diuretics have been used for many years to treat hypertension, but they have not been used to reduce coronary mortality post-myocardial infarction (MI) and they have not been considered as cardioprotective drugs. However, three studies[1-3] in which thiazides were given to elderly hypertensives produced a reduction in coronary mortality. These results and other factors have persuaded national and international groups who advise on the treatment of hypertension to suggest that thiazide diuretics or beta-blockers should be the first-line treatment for hypertension. Since the main reason for treating hypertension is to prevent coronary and cerebrovascular events, we need to consider briefly the evidence that they reduce the risk of having a coronary event. The capacity to reduce the risk of suffering from cerebrovascular disease is well established and not doubted.[1-3]

Mechanisms
There is little or no evidence that thiazide diuretics reduce endothelial damage, atheroma formation, clot formation or reduce the risk of ventricular fibrillation (VF). On the contrary,

the increases in plasma glucose, lipids, uric acid and viscosity would be expected to increase the risk of coronary occlusive disease and the tendency to lower plasma potassium and magnesium would be expected to increase the risk of VF.[4,5]

Primary prevention trials

Prior to 1985 several trials including a major Veteran Administration Study (1970)[6] and the Australian trial (1979)[7] compared diuretics with placebo. These studies tended to show a marked reduction in the number of cerebrovascular events but the impact on coronary events was small and non significant. McMahon and colleagues[8,9] analysed the data and drew attention to the relative lack of impact of blood pressure reduction usually with thiazide diuretics on CAD mortality. Thus a blood pressure reduction which brought the pressure to a level which would have been expected to lower coronary event rate by 20–25% and was associated with a 20–25% lower stroke rate only produced an 8–12% reduction in coronary events[8,9].

The MRC (1985) trial[10] showed that the coronary events in men on thiazides and on placebo were identical and in the MAPHY trial[11,12] whilst metoprolol and thiazides had the same impact on stroke, the coronary mortality was higher on thiazide diuretics.

There are also studies[13–15] which have associated diuretic therapy with an increased risk of sudden death, a major contribution to the total mortality from coronary disease. The study by Siscovick and colleagues[14] also showed that the risk of sudden deaths was dose related and that the combination of low dose thiazide diuretic with a potassium sparing diuretic reduced the risk (see Table 1). The addition of potassium supplements did not seem to help. These observations may help to explain the better results in more recent trials in which lower doses of thiazides are used and are often given with potassium sparing diuretics.

It is against this background that the three studies[1–3] in the elderly have to be considered. The SHEP trial[2] (Systolic Hypertension in the Elderly Programme) included those with systolic hypertension and the main initial therapy was chlorthalidone without a potassium sparing diuretic. The coronary mortality was reduced from 26 (out of 2371) on placebo to 15 (out of 2362) on active therapy. The sudden death numbers were 44 and 47 for active and placebo therapy respectively. In the STOP-hypertension

	Odds ratio	95% CI
100 mg Thiazide	2.4	0.7–8.0
50 mg Thiazide	1.1	0.5–2.5
25 mg Thiazide	0.7	0.2–2.5
50 mg Thiazide plus PSD	0.5	0.1–2.2
25 mg Thiazide plus PSD	0.3	0.1–1.0

Table 2.1 The risk of primary cardiac arrest expressed as odds ratio (with 95 per cent confidence intervals) for different doses of thiazide (hydrochlorathiazide or chlorthalidone) and thiazides in combination with potassium-sparing diuretic (PSD). Adapted from Siscovick et al[14].

trial[3] the patients were either on thiazide diuretics with potassium sparing diuretics or beta-blockers and the results on each treatment were not reported separately making it impossible to comment specifically on the impact of diuretics. In the MRC elderly trial[1] the patients were randomized to atenolol, hydrochlorothiazide 25mg plus amiloride 5mg or placebo. In this study the coronary mortality was reduced on the diuretics (diuretics 5.2, atenolol 8.2, placebo 8.6 per 1000 patient years). Sudden death rates were not reported.

Secondary prevention
No data available

Conclusion
Diuretics lower blood pressure and this is associated with some reduction in coronary events. In most early studies the impact was small and usually not significant. The most impressive result was the MRC Elderly study in which diuretics reduced the coronary event rates by 2.4 per 1000 patient years.

This result is supported by the data from the other recent studies in the elderly.

Diuretic therapy is being very actively encouraged as first line therapy for hypertension. This is largely based on the results of three studies in the elderly and is an endorsement of low dose therapy with a potassium sparing diuretic. However, prescribers should note the metabolic effects of higher doses of thiazides, the modest impact of thiazides in earlier studies on younger populations and the association of thiazide therapy with an increased risk of sudden death.

■ BETA-ADRENOCEPTOR BLOCKING DRUGS (BETA-BLOCKERS)

Beta-blockers probably come closest to meeting the criteria for being accepted as cardioprotective drugs. However, the available evidence is confusing because not all beta-blockers are equally effective and because, with the benefit of hindsight, primary prevention trials were not well designed. Nevertheless a case can be made that beta-blockers, and perhaps especially lipophilic beta-blockers, are cardioprotective; they have an impact on the pathological processes leading to death from coronary disease, and there are clinical trial data that (1) suggest a role in primary prevention, (2) show an impact at the time of infarction, and (3) provide clear evidence of secondary prevention.

☐ Mechanisms

Endothelial injury

Haemodynamic factors cause endothelial damage and determine the sites of injury and subsequent atheroma formation. High blood pressure,[16,17] tachycardia[18] and a stressed personality[19] predispose to coronary disease, and atheromatous lesions tend to form at sites of wall stress and high turbulence.[20,21] Beta-blockers lower blood pressure, reduce heart rate, reduce peripheral responses to stress and counteract the tendency for lesions to form at branching sites in arteries.[22] Although several investigators have used different models to study the impact of beta-blockers on endothelial damage, the experiments of Kaplan and colleagues on stressed monkeys are most relevant.[23,24] Dominant monkeys became stressed if they were required to keep establishing their dominance over other monkeys when moved from group to group. Such animals develop endothelial damage which may be prevented by either propranolol[23] or metoprolol.[24] Spence et al[25] provided further evidence by assessing the effects of hypertension and a high-cholesterol diet on rabbits. Propranolol was much more effective than hydralazine in reducing the aortic surface area affected by atheroma.

Atheroma formation
There is some evidence to suggest that most antihypertensive drugs can reduce atheroma formation. The data on beta-blockers are more extensive and more impressive.[26,27] Kaplan et al[26] reviewed 13 studies, in 11 of which beta-blockers (mostly propranolol) reduced atheroma formation in animals. The impact of beta-blockers was not related to blood pressure reduction and occurred despite small adverse effects on plasma lipids. It is not yet clear how beta-blockers achieve their effects but it is probably partly by reducing lipid binding to damaged endothelium,[22] and to arterial wall proteoglycans.[28]

Plaque rupture
There are no data to support the belief that the risk of plaque rupture may be reduced by decreasing the haemodynamic strains imposed by high blood pressure and rapid heart rates. Nevertheless, it seems a reasonable hypothesis that beta-blockers may reduce the risk.[29]

Clot formation
Beta-blockers may reduce platelet aggregation,[30,31] increase prostacyclin formation[32] and favourably modify the fibrinolytic system.[33]

Infarction size
The consensus view is that beta-blockers reduce infarction size. Studies that have failed to show this effect have often been performed on unsuitable laboratory animal models or beta-blockers were given too late. There is a substantial quantity of animal data[34] but the most impressive information comes from large-scale human studies.[35–38]

Ventricular fibrillation
Ventricular fibrillation (VF) tends to occur when myocardial ischaemia is associated with high sympathetic drive and low vagal

tone.[39] Beta-blockers do have anti-ischaemic effects as set out above and do protect from the effects of sympathetic drive. Until recently, the possibility that lipophilic beta-blockers may have an effect on vagal tone by an action on autonomic centres in the brain was not appreciated. There are now data to show that low doses of propranolol given into the cerebral ventricles reduce the risk of VF in a stressed-pig model.[40] It has also been shown that in the dog with left ventricular hypertrophy, blood pressure reduction with metoprolol but not with enalapril reduces the risk of VF in response to acute coronary occlusion.[41] Finally, in a rabbit model rendered vulnerable by chloralose anaesthesia and acute coronary occlusion, metoprolol, but not atenolol, reduced the risk of VF[42] (Figure 2.1). The effect of metoprolol was shown to be related to its capacity to increase vagal tone.[42] These three animal models demonstrating the effects of beta-blockers are of considerable interest, though their relevance to human beings is open to question. Nevertheless, they help to explain the impact

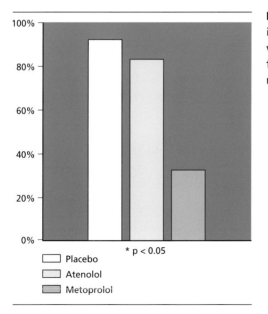

Figure 2.1 The incidence of ventricular fibrillation (%) in rabbits.[42]

Patient type	Name	Year of publication	Drugs used	Impact on coronary mortality
Middle-aged	MRC	1988	Thiazide Propranolol	None
	IPPPSH	1985	Oxprenolol	Reduced in non-smoking males
	HAPPHY	1985	Atenolol/metoprolol Thiazide	None
	MAPHY	1987	Metoprolol Thiazide	Decreased
Elderly	Coope and Warrender		Atenolol/diuretic Placebo	None
	STOP	1992	Beta-blocker/thiazide Placebo	Reduced
	MRC Elderly	1992	Atenolol Placebo Thiazide	None Reduced

Table 2.2 Primary prevention trials.

on sudden death in one primary prevention trial,[43] in three secondary prevention trials[36,44,45] and in two clinical studies on the incidence of VF.[46,47]

☐ Clinical data

Primary prevention

There have been three major primary prevention trials in middle-aged hypertensives and three trials in the elderly (Table 2.2) which have assessed the impact of beta-blockade. Data on total mortality are presented in Figure 2.2. Coronary events and sudden deaths are presented in Figure 2.3.

MRC (1985) Trial[10]

The aim of this trial was to compare the effects of propranolol, a thiazide diuretic, and placebo on middle-aged hypertensives of either sex; 17 354 patients were entered into the study. The overall rates for coronary events per 1000 patient years were propranolol 4.8, bendrofluazide 5.6, and placebo 5.5. These results were not significantly different from each other; in relation to coronary disease this trial was judged to have had a negative result. It did not produce evidence to support the belief that a beta-blocker would reduce the coronary event rate.

Unfortunately the MRC trial had three main defects. First, since there was a placebo group, the patient population had mild hypertension (diastolic blood pressure 90–109 mmHg). It would have been unethical to deny active treatment to anyone with more severe hypertension. However, 18 per cent of placebo patients were normotensive on their first three annual visits and many more were intermittently normotensive. It is difficult to demonstrate a coronary preventive effect by modifying one risk factor that was only present in a proportion of patients. Second, about half the population was female. In this group the risk of a coronary event was about 1.7 per 1000 patient years and this risk was halved in non-smokers. It is difficult to demonstrate a reduction in the risk of coronary events below 0.8 per 1000 patient years. Finally, a minority of major coronary events are easily recognized. To assess the impact of treatment, good data on overt coronary events, silent infarctions and all sudden cardiac deaths are needed. In a post-hoc analysis, with all the potential for bias that this entails, propranolol did reduce the risk of

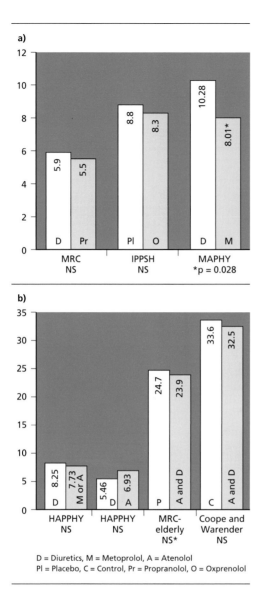

Figure 2.2 Total mortality rates per 1000 patient years: (a) propranolol, oxprenolol and metoprolol, (b) atenolol studies. D = diuretics; M = metoprolol; A = atenolol; Pl = placebo; C = control; Pr = propranolol; O = oxprenolol.
*Atenolol alone 26.4

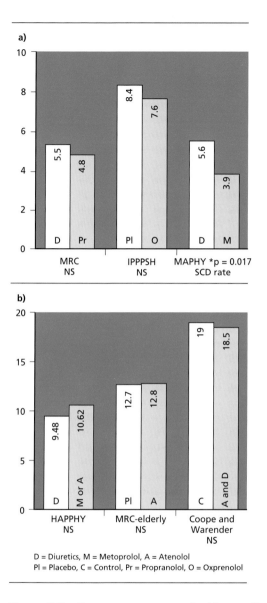

Figure 2.3 Coronary events rate (sudden cardiac death, non-fatal MI: (a) propranolol, oxprenolol and metoprolol, (b) atenolol studies. D = diuretics; Pr = propranolol; O = oxprenolol; M = metoprolol; A = atenolol; C = control; Pl = placebo.

cardiovascular events in non-smokers and, when silent infarctions were included,[48] propranolol did significantly reduce the coronary event rate.

The IPPPSH trial[49]

The International Prospective Primary Prevention Study in Hypertension aimed to compare an antihypertensive regimen based on the beta-blocker oxprenolol with one not containing a beta-blocker in a population of mild-to-moderately hypertensive men and women. This trial failed to yield a clear-cut result but, like the MRC trial, the beta-blocker regimen was associated with fewer cardiac events in men. In male non-smokers the impact on critical cardiac events (5.4 versus 11.5 per 1000 patient years) in favour of oxprenolol was impressive. However, dredging data in this way may be misleading and it is noteworthy that females seemed to fare less well on oxprenolol.

The HAPPHY-MAPHY Trial[11,50]

This trial has been a major source of controversy and its findings have not been accepted by many. However, the results of later studies and other investigations lend some support to its original conclusions.

The trial was originally devised in 1977 as a comparison between metoprolol and a thiazide in males with moderate hypertension. By 1979 atenolol had become available and therefore other centres were recruited in which atenolol was compared with a thiazide in the belief that the two cardioselective beta-blockers would behave similarly. In 1985, at a time when some of the atenolol centre patients had only been in the trial a short time, it was decided to analyse the results combining the atenolol and metoprolol data and comparing them with the thiazide results from all centres. Overall, beta-blockers did not reduce either total mortality (Figure 2.2) or coronary events (Figure 2.3) when compared with thiazides.[50] It therefore seemed to be a negative trial and thus, taken in conjunction with the overall results of the MRC and IPPPSH trials, strongly suggested that beta-blockers were not cardioprotective.

Following the initial analysis and without knowing the results for the individual beta-blockers, a controversial decision was made that the metoprolol/thiazide centres would continue to recruit and to monitor the progress of their patients. Many at the time regarded this as totally unacceptable. However, these data were subsequently published as the MAPHY trial and showed that metoprolol reduced overall mortality, coronary mortality,[11] sudden deaths[43] and coronary morbidity.[12]

Many found it inexplicable and therefore unacceptable that metoprolol should seem to be cardioprotective though atenolol was not. In addition, most regarded the notion of continuing to monitor one subgroup after an initial analysis had been performed as not abiding by the rules of clinical trial methodology. Nevertheless, subsequent data have not shown that atenolol is cardioprotective.[1,51] Fierce arguments against[52,53] and in favour of[54,55] the MAPHY trial have been presented.

Trials in the elderly

Trials of primary prevention in the elderly contribute little to this subject and merit brief mention. Coope and Warrender[56] showed that it was worth treating elderly hypertensives with atenolol alone or with a diuretic to reduce the risk of stroke, but there was little impact on coronary mortality. The SHEP trial[2] evaluated the role of a thiazide diuretic to which atenolol could be added in patients with isolated systolic hypertension. It showed that antihypertensive therapy very effectively reduced stroke risk but also showed that most cardiovascular deaths are due to coronary disease (132/202) and many (91/202) are sudden deaths. These latter are not reduced by thiazides (with or without atenolol).

In the STOP-Hypertension trial,[3] elderly patients with hypertension were given either a beta-blocker (80 per cent) or a diuretic. Beta-blockers included metoprolol, atenolol and pindolol. Treatment reduced total mortality but also seemed to reduce coronary mortality and sudden death. In the MRC (elderly) trial,[1] although active treatment reduced the risk of stroke, atenolol did not have an impact on coronary disease.

In conclusion, although the primary prevention data on beta-blockers are unsatisfactory for several reasons, in the groups that are especially vulnerable, namely middle-aged hypertensive men, a lipophilic beta-blocker may have beneficial effects on coronary mortality[10,11,48,49] (see Figures 2.2 and 2.3) whereas atenolol had little impact[1,51,56] (see Figures 2.2b and 2.3b).

Secondary prevention

Beta-blockers have been given both acutely and long term. In the former case the drug is usually given intravenously within a few hours of onset of symptoms suggestive of MI. Treatment may be continued for a few days or a few weeks. Long-term therapy is given orally and continued for months or even years.

Acute studies

Many small studies and two large trials have been performed.[57] In ISIS-1,[58] 16 105 patients were randomized to receive atenolol or placebo. Atenolol reduced mortality significantly by about 14 per cent, the impact being mainly during the initial 24–48 h post-MI and due in large measure to a reduction in cardiac rupture. In the other large study, the MIAMI trial,[59] 5778 patients were randomized to either metoprolol or placebo. The overall reduction in mortality was comparable (13 per cent) but this was not statistically significant; the effect was not limited to the initial 1–2 days and was most marked in the patients at greater risk.[59] The results of these trials are summarized in Figure 2.4.

Chronic studies

Over 50 000 individuals have been entered into trials designed to assess the effects of chronic beta-blockade in post-MI patients. The benefits of beta-blockers are well known, although their use is not as widespread as might be expected.

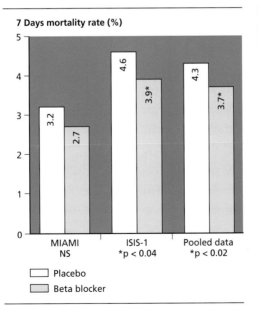

Figure 2.4 Acute post-MI beta-blocker studies.

- The Norwegian Timolol Study[44] was a landmark clinical trial; 4155 patients from a catchment population equivalent to one-third of Norway were enrolled 6–27 days post-MI. The study was double blind and the patients were followed for a mean 17 months. Of the patients, 184 died either whilst on treatment or within 28 days of withdrawal. Of the deaths, 93 per cent were cardiac and 77 per cent were sudden. Timolol reduced total mortality (Figure 2.5) and cardiac mortality, and dramatically reduced the rates for sudden death by 44.6 per cent ($P = 0.0001$) (Figure 2.6). It also reduced reinfarction rates. The positive effects on sudden death were maintained through the study and infarction rates were reduced over at least the first 6 months. Furthermore, not only did older patients – i.e. those aged 65–75 years – tolerate the treatment, but also those on active therapy had a lower mortality ($n = 28$ versus $n = 9$) and a lower infarction rate ($n = 33$ versus $n = 69$).

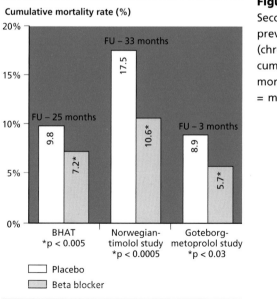

Figure 2.5 Secondary prevention (chronic studies): cumulative mortality (%). FU = mean follow-up.

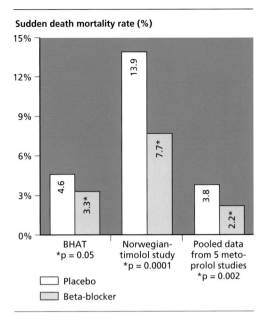

Figure 2.6
Secondary prevention (chronic studies): sudden cardiac death mortality rate (%).

Sudden death mortality rate (%)

BHAT
*p = 0.05

Norwegian-timolol study
*p = 0.0001

Pooled data from 5 metoprolol studies
*p = 0.002

Placebo

Beta-blocker

- The Gothenberg Metoprolol Trial[36] differed from the Norwegian trial in that the study lasted for 3 months but in this case the beta-blocker (metoprolol) was given intravenously as soon as possible after admission. The study included 1395 patients, and 40 (5.7 per cent) on metoprolol and 62 (8.9 per cent) on placebo died, a significant difference. Beta-blocker therapy reduced total mortality (Figure 2.5) and had a striking impact on sudden death, with a substantial reduction in episodes of VF. Metoprolol was well tolerated. The beneficial effect on sudden death has been confirmed in other studies[60] (Figure 2.6).
- The Beta-blocker Heart Attack Trial (BHAT)[45] was a large US study in which 3837 patients were given propranolol or placebo, starting on average 13 days post-MI with a mean follow-up of 25 months. Again, mortality (7.2 per cent versus 9.8 per cent) (Figure 2.5) and sudden death (3.3 per cent versus 4.6 per cent) (Figure 2.6) were significantly diminished.

The above trials and others involving many thousands of patients have demonstrated convincingly that in post-MI patients beta-blocker therapy increases the chances of survival by 20–40 per cent.[61–63] In particular, beta-blockers reduce the risk of sudden death.[64] However, in spite of this scientific evidence, the use of beta-blockers in clinical practice is relatively low.[61,63,65] Thus a recent review of elderly post-MI patients determined which patients would have been eligible to receive beta-blockers. Of those who were eligible, only 21 per cent were actually given a beta-blocker but, after controlling for all other risk predictors, those put on a beta-blocker had a mortality rate 43 per cent less than those who were not given a beta-blocker.[63] Use of a calcium channel blocker instead of a beta-blocker doubled the risk. Further, in the CAST study[66] the anti-arrhythmic drugs did not reduce mortality, but in a retrospective study it was noted that those patients in the CAST study who were on a beta-blocker did have a significantly lower mortality rate.[67]

Patients with diabetes mellitus

Diabetic patients are at considerably increased risk of having an MI and of dying from it. This is discussed in Chapter 3. However, since many regard diabetes as a relative contraindication to the use of beta-blockers, the beneficial impact of beta-blockers based on four post-MI studies, as described by Kjekshus et al[68] and demonstrated in Figure 2.7, merits emphasis in this section.

A recent report of an observational study[69] described a 3-year follow-up of non-insulin-dependent diabetics known to have CAD who were originally documented as part of a screening programme to identify suitable patients for the Bezafibrate Infarction Prevention (BIP) Study. Of the patients, 911 (33 per cent) were on a beta-blocker and had a mortality rate of 7.8 per cent, and 1812 (67 per cent) were not on a beta-blocker and their mortality rate was 14 per cent. Though this was not a randomized trial, these results do suggest an association between beta-blocker therapy and improved survival.

Conclusion

Some of the data on beta-blockers have proved controversial. However, overall the data on mechanisms and the primary and the secondary prevention data provide unequivocal evidence that beta-blockers are cardioprotective, the post-MI data being the most persuasive.[70] Interestingly but controversially, the evidence suggests that it is the lipophilic beta-blockers which are cardioprotective.

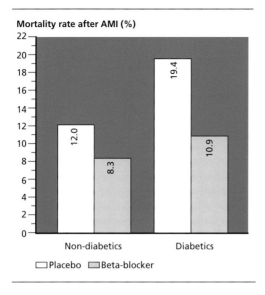

Mortality rate after AMI (%)

Non-diabetics: Placebo 12.0, Beta-blocker 8.3
Diabetics: Placebo 19.4, Beta-blocker 10.9

☐ Placebo   ☐ Beta-blocker

Figure 2.7
Combined data on the impact of beta-blockers on mortality post-MI in non-diabetics and in diabetics.[68]

■ CALCIUM ANTAGONISTS

Calcium antagonists are used extensively in the management of angina and hypertension, conditions which indicate that the patient already has or is likely to develop CAD. However, though these drugs have antiatherogenic, vasodilator and antiarrhythmic properties, most clinical trials have failed to show any capacity to reduce the incidence of or mortality from CAD. There is even evidence from a number of sources to suggest that some calcium antagonists (short-acting dihydropyridines) may increase coronary mortality,[71–73] though this has been disputed.[74] Though the matter remains contentious;[75] regulatory authorities and prescribing doctors have responded to recent publications by deciding that short-acting dihydropyridines should not be used in the treatment of hypertension, in unstable angina or in the early days after an MI (except when given with a beta-blocker).

A recent observational study suggests that longer-acting dihydropyridines do not increase the risk of a coronary event,[76] though further information from proper randomized trials will be required to establish the safety of the long acting preparations.[77]

Calcium antagonists, or slow calcium channel blocking drugs, all have some effect on peripheral arteries, myocardial contractility and the cardiac conducting tissues. However, the different types of calcium antagonist differ in their impact on different tissues. The potential effects on mechanisms are considered for the group as a whole but the clinical actions of the dihydropyridines (nifedipine-like drugs) the phenylalkylamines (e.g. verapamil) and the benzothiazepines (e.g. diltiazem) will be considered separately.

Mechanisms

Calcium antagonists have been shown to have some impact on many of the processes that lead to the development of an infarct and to death from arrhythmias. Their potential to reduce atheroma formation and to encourage its regression has been a subject of particular interest. However, not all calcium antagonists are the same. Some may have a useful cardioprotective role as suggested by their actions described below.

Atheroma formation

Calcium deposition is a well established part of the process leading to atheroma formation.[78,79] The more extensive the disease the higher the calcium content, and the greater the amount of calcium the greater the loss of the capacity to expand and contract in response to prevailing pressures.[80] Reducing calcium deposition retards the development of atheroma.[81]

In the classic model, the cholesterol-fed rabbit, most types of calcium antagonist reduce aortic atheroma formation.[82] Nifedipine has a striking effect and isradipine is even more effective.[82] It is not clear how this benefit is achieved but possible mechanisms include reducing endothelial permeability[83] or calcium overload. These drugs may also increase cholesterol ester removal by stimulating cholesteryl ester hydrolase, modifying LDL receptors, or inhibiting matrix component synthesis and smooth muscle cell migration and proliferation.[82] All these actions are achieved independently of an antihypertensive effect of the calcium antagonist and without altering plasma lipid concentrations. Furthermore, they exert their preventive effect very early in the development of atheroma.[83,84] Calcium antagonists seem unable to delay progression of atherogenesis once it has advanced beyond the early stages.

Clot formation

Calcium antagonists reduce platelet aggregation[85] but there is little evidence of any change in susceptibility to clot formation.

Data from experimental coronary occlusion studies have shown that calcium antagonists reduce infarction size. The impact will depend on the nature of the coronary circulation of the animal studied, timing of the drug dosing in relation to the coronary occlusion, the properties of the particular calcium antagonist and the methods used to determine infarction size.[86,87] Dihydropyridines (particularly nifedipine), verapamil and diltiazem have all been shown to reduce infarction size.[88]

Ventricular fibrillation

Calcium antagonists, notably verapamil, are effective in the management of supraventricular tachycardias, but have little or no impact on serious ventricular arrhythmias.

☐ Dihydropyridines

Primary prevention

There are no convincing data to suggest that patients with either hypertension or angina are less likely to have an MI or to die if they are being treated with a dihydropyridine calcium antagonist. They may even be at marginally greater risk.[71–73] However, there are studies suggesting that this group of drugs may have a positive beneficial effect on the progression of CAD.

Loaldi et al[89] reported a study on angina patients treated with nifedipine, propranolol or isosorbide dinitrate (ISDN). The progression of pre-existing lesions over a 2-year period occurred in 31 per cent on nifedipine, 53 per cent on propranolol and 47 per cent on ISDN. Furthermore, the appearance of new lesions was lower on nifedipine (10 per cent) compared with propranolol (34 per cent) and ISDN (29 per cent).

The INTACT (International Nifedipine Trial on Atherosclerosis Therapy) study was designed to assess the impact of nifedipine on the progression of CAD.[90] In this relatively long-term, randomized, double-blind trial, 425 patients with mild

CAD had angiographic studies before and after a 3-year course of treatment. Computer-assisted measurements showed no significant difference in the number, severity or progression of pre-existing lesions, but the number of new lesions per patient was significantly fewer in those on nifedipine (28 per cent reduction). During the study, active therapy did not influence the frequency of non-fatal MIs, the severity of unstable angina or the need for revascularization procedures. However, there were more cardiac deaths in those on nifedipine (8:2) (Figure 2.8).

The Montreal Heart Institute Study (MHIS)[91] was conducted as a double-blind placebo-controlled study in 383 patients (with 5–75 per cent stenoses in at least four coronary artery segments) treated with nicardipine or placebo. Coronary arteriography was

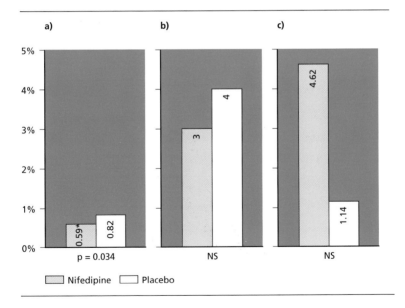

Figure 2.8 Results of the intact study: (a) number (%) of new lesions per patient: (b) regression of pre-existing lesions (%); (c) cardiac death rate.

repeated at 24 months in 335 patients. Mean progression and regression of single lesions and of disease in individual patients were comparable on nicardipine or placebo. But there was a significantly lower rate of progression of minor-grade stenoses (<20 per cent of luminal narrowings) in the nicardipine group compared with placebo (15 per cent versus 27 per cent of patients). Cardiac death was distributed equally between nicardipine and placebo groups, but MI occurred more often among patients on nicardipine than placebo (14 patients with 17 MIs in the nicardipine group versus eight patients with nine MIs in the placebo group).

Secondary prevention

Acute effects
Eight trials assessed the impact of nifedipine given acutely after an MI.[92–99] Seven reported mortality rates that are presented in Figure 2.9 and Table 2.3; the eighth[97] reported on the progression of patients with angina and threatened infarction.

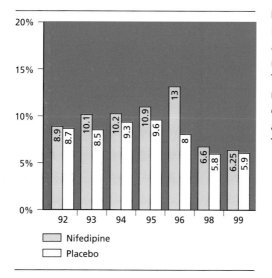

Figure 2.9
Mortality rate (%), acute post-MI nifedipine studies. The authors and references for each of the seven trials are present in Table 2.3.

Study	Nifedipine	Placebo	Statistical significance
Sirens et al[92]	8.9	8.7	NS
Muller et al[93]	10.1	8.5	NS
Wilcox et al[94]	10.2	9.3	NS
Branagan et al[95]	10.9	9.6	NS
Erbel et al[96]	13.0	8.0	NS
Walker et al[98]	6.6	5.8	NS
Gotlieb et al[99]	6.25	5.9	NS

Table 2.3 Mortality rate (%), acute post-MI nifedipine studies.

The Norwegian Nifedipine Multicenter Trial[92] included 272 patients with the diagnosis of suspected MI seen within 12 h of the onset of symptoms. Definite MI developed in 67 per cent of the nifedipine patients and in 73 per cent of the patients receiving placebo, which was not a significant difference. Infarction size was similar in both groups, as was mortality after 6 weeks.

In the Nifedipine–Threatened and Acute Myocardial Infarction Study,[93] 105 patients with threatened MI and 66 patients with acute MI (AMI) were included and treated with nifedipine a mean of 4.6 h after the onset of symptoms. Nifedipine did not reduce the likelihood of progression from threatened MI to AMI, since 75 per cent of each group (nifedipine and placebo) went on to infarct. Infarction size was also similar in both groups. Two-week mortality was 7.9 per cent in the nifedipine group and 0 per cent in the placebo group. This finding raises the possibility that nifedipine exacerbated the sequelae of infarction. There was no difference in total mortality at 6 months (10.1 per cent nifedipine; 8.5 per cent placebo).

The Trial of Early Nifedipine Treatment (TRENT) studied 4491 patients with suspected MI.[94] Within 24 h of the onset of symptoms, patients received treatment with oral nifedipine. In both groups, 64 per cent of patients developed an AMI during the observation period. The mortality rate in patients with confirmed MI was 10.2 per cent in the treated group versus 9.3 per cent in the placebo group. Compared with the placebo group, the nifedipine-treated patients were found to have significant decreases in systolic and diastolic pressure and increases in heart rate.[94]

Branagan et al[95] conducted a study that included 98 patients with suspected MI who received nifedipine or placebo approximately 3.3 h from the onset of symptoms. There were no significant differences in one-month mortality or infarction size between the two groups. Also, there was no significant difference at 1 month in the progression from the coronary insufficiency to MI.

Erbel et al[96] reported the results of a trial in 149 patients with chest pain lasting longer than 30 min, together with ECG changes, who received either nifedipine or placebo treatment immediately. All patients were given intracoronary streptokinase and, in addition, the nifedipine group were given intracoronary nifedipine before and after the thrombolytic therapy. The in-hospital mortality rate was 13 per cent in the nifedipine group and 8 per cent in the placebo group. Patients treated with nifedipine had 16 per cent incidence of reinfarction versus 11 per cent in the placebo group. Reocclusion of the infarct-related vessel occurred in 20 per cent of the nifedipine group and in 13 per cent of the patients in the placebo group. None of the reported differences were significant.

Although not significant, this trend towards increased cardiovascular morbidity and mortality in nifedipine-treated patients is disturbing (Table 2.3; Figure 2.9). In other acute MI trials with nifedipine, there were no significant differences between nifedipine and placebo group with respect to infarction size, the incidence of ventricular arrhythmias or hospital mortality.[97–99]

Long-term effects (Table 2.4 and Figure 2.10)

The Secondary Prevention Reinfarction Israeli Nifedipine Trial (SPRINT 1)[100] included 2276 patients 7–21 days after AMI. They were randomized to receive nifedipine or placebo for a mean duration of 10 months. The 10–month mortality rate in the placebo group was 5.75 per cent versus 5.8 per cent in the nifedipine-treated group. There was no difference in recurrent MI between the nifedipine and placebo groups (4.4 per cent versus 4.8 per cent respectively). The authors concluded that nifedipine beginning 2 or 3 weeks after the event does not reduce mortality or recurrent infarction.

Study	Nifedipine	Placebo	Statistical significance
SPRINT I[100]	5.8	5.7	NS
SPRINT II[101]	9.3	9.3	NS

Table 2.4 Mortality rate (%), long-term nifedipine studies.

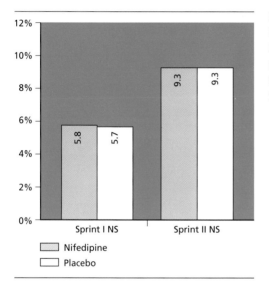

Figure 2.10
Mortality rate (%).
Long-term
nifedipine studies:
SPRINT I[100] and
SPRINT II.[101]

In the placebo-controlled SPRINT II trial,[101] 1373 patients were randomized to receive nifedipine as soon as possible after the onset of AMI. Follow-up was 6 months. There was no difference in mortality between the two groups (9.3 per cent in both). But mortality was higher in nifedipine-treated patients who initially presented with low systolic blood pressure (<100 mmHg). Thus, SPRINT II extended the preliminary conclusion of SPRINT I that neither early nor late administration of nifedipine has any effect in subsequent cardiac events in survivors of MI.

Despite many theoretical reasons, some animal data, and angiographic evidence of benefit, clinical studies have failed to show a benefit from calcium antagonist treatment. Long-term primary prevention studies in hypertension have not been performed and short-term studies in unstable angina or acutely post-MI have been negative.[71] Longer term post-infarct studies have not demonstrated any reduction in reinfarction or mortality.

Further in the MIDAS trial isradipine or hydrochlorathiazide were given in a randomized double blind trial to assess their impact on intimal to medial thickness in carotid arteries.[102] There was no difference in changes in the carotid walls but vascular events (MI, stroke, CCF, sudden death, angina) were more frequent in those on isradipine. The lack of impact in the acute setting might be attributed to the vasodilatation that stimulates an increase in sympathetic nervous system activity and which is potentially counterproductive. This could be controlled by giving a dihydropyridine with a beta-blocker; there is some evidence for this notion.[97]

Recent concerns about dihydropyridines

The evidence for the lack of any positive impact on CAD has been apparent for some time and was clearly set out in a review by Held et al.[71] Their review included information on all types of calcium antagonists derived from 22 trials in which 19 100 patients had been entered. They noted that the mortality rate on nifedipine was 7.7 per cent (365 out of 4731 patients) compared with 7.0 per cent (330 out of 4733) on placebo.

More recently the results of an observational study by Psaty and colleagues[72] has provoked considerable interest. The patients from Puget Sound, Seattle, all had hypertension and were on treatment. Between 1986 and 1993, patients who had their first fatal or non fatal MI (cases) were matched with 2032 treated hypertensives who did not have an MI. Using diuretic therapy as their comparator, they found that those on short-acting calcium channel blockers were more likely to have an MI (risk ratio 1.62, 95 per cent CI 1.11–2.34: $P = 0.01$). Furthermore, the higher the dose, the greater the risk. This observation has provoked a number of publications and public confrontations which have attempted to confirm or refute the evidence.[74,75] This matter has been the subject of considerable controversy but the lack of evidence for a beneficial effect of short-acting dihydropyridines on CAD risk and the suspicions of a small increase in risk have led some regulatory authorities to suggest that there is a very limited role for these drugs.

There is no evidence against the long-acting dihydropyridines and a good observational study reported by Alderman and colleagues[76] is reassuring, but further data are needed.[77] The recently published Syst-Eur study offers one indication that calcium channel blockers are safe and effective in an elderly, relatively fit population.[77a] Among patients over 60 years old with isolated systolic hypertension, a treatment regimen including nitrendipine significantly reduced rates of stroke, the primary end point.

☐ Verapamil

Primary prevention

Verapamil is a calcium antagonist with definite antiarrhythmic properties which has been shown to have useful antiatherogenic actions in animal studies and tends to increase plasma concentrations of high-density lipoproteins (HDL) in humans[103]. However, as yet there is no good evidence that it will reduce the risk of having an MI or dying from it. There is some evidence that it has a beneficial impact on atheroma formation in humans.

In the Frankfurt retrospective trial,[104] a group of 43 patients aged 40–65 years with CAD was evaluated. After the initial angiography, 26 patients received long-term therapy with verapamil and 17 patients received conventional antianginal therapy (beta-blockers and nitrates). Average follow-up was 13 months. Coronary lesions regressed in a significantly greater proportion of patients on verapamil (21 per cent) than in patients on standard therapy (8 per cent). Regression of high-grade stenosis (41 per cent) occurred significantly more frequently than regression of low-grade stenoses (12 per cent) in the verapamil group.

A prospective study, the Frankfurt Isoptin Progression Study (FIPS),[83] involved 445 patients after coronary artery bypass surgery (i.e. advanced stages of CAD) who were randomized to either verapamil or placebo. Angiographic evaluations were performed 3 years after enrolment in 79 patients on verapamil and 80 patients on placebo. No significant differences were found between the two groups with regard to progression or regression of pre-existing stenoses, development of new stenoses or new occlusions in either the native vessels or in bypass grafts. There were no differences in progression or regression of stenoses of low or high grade between treatment groups. Cardiac deaths (five in the verapamil group and three in the placebo group) and the need for bypass surgery were equally distributed between both groups.

The Verapamil in Hypertension Atherosclerosis Study (VHAS) is an ongoing study designed to compare verapamil slow release and chlorthalidone in lowering blood pressure, retarding atherosclerotic progression in carotid arteries in hypertensive patients and reducing cardiovascular mortality.[105] The double-blind, 3-year study includes 1464 patients with essential hypertension.

Secondary prevention

Acute effects
Crea and colleagues[106] reported the results of a single-blind placebo-controlled study in 17 patients with AMI. They were given verapamil or placebo in an intravenous regimen. Treatment was started a mean of 6.5 h after the onset of symptoms. The study failed to prevent angina and reinfarction in patients after AMI.

The only clinical trial reporting any benefit from verapamil given early in an AMI was conducted by Bussman et al.[107] They included 54 patients treated with intravenous verapamil. A reduction of 30 per cent in creatine kinase, the cardiac isoenzyme (CK-MB) release was observed. The group on verapamil required less lignocaine and diuretic therapy than the control group. This small study was not double blind.

Long-term studies
Based on the evidence of experimental studies in which verapamil has been shown to reduce infarction size, the Danish study group conducted a randomized, placebo-controlled, double-blind trial: the Danish Verapamil Infarction Trial (DAVIT-1)[108]. The aim was to determine whether an intravenous bolus of verapamil followed by oral verapamil for 6 months might decrease total death and reinfarction rate. DAVIT-I included 717 patients in the verapamil group and 719 patients in the placebo group. The differences in mortality and reinfarction rates between the two groups after 6 months were not significant.

Retrospective analysis of the data showed a lower mortality rate in the verapamil group (3.7 per cent) versus placebo group (6.4 per cent) between days 22 and 180. The reinfarction rate was 3.9 per cent in the verapamil group compared with 7.0 per cent in the placebo group between days 15 and 180.[108] These results encouraged the authors to conduct a late intervention trial to investigate whether the treatment with verapamil from the second week after an AMI, continued for at least 1 year, might reduce total mortality and major events (cardiac death and reinfarction).

The Danish Verapamil Infarction Trial II (DAVIT-II)[109] was also a double-blind placebo-controlled multicentre study that included 878 patients on verapamil and 897 patients on placebo started in the second week after admission to the hospital and continued for a mean of 16 months. The 18-month cumulative mortality rate was 11.2 per cent and 13.8 per cent in the verapamil and placebo groups, respectively. The sudden death rate was 5.7 per cent and 7.5 per cent and the cardiac death rate was 9.9 per cent and 12.3 per cent in the verapamil group and placebo groups, respectively. These differences were not significant. However, there were 91 reinfarctions on verapamil compared with 129 in the placebo group. The 18-month first reinfarction rate was 11 per cent in the verapamil group and 13.2 per cent in placebo group (Figure 2.11). In patients without heart

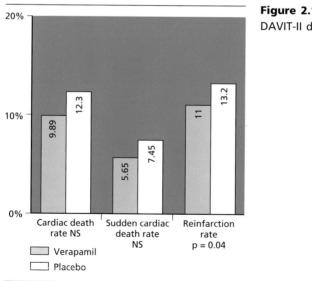

Figure 2.11
DAVIT-II data.[109]

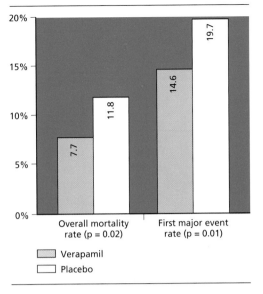

Figure 2.12
DAVIT-II – patients
without heart
failure[109]

Overall mortality
rate (p = 0.02)

First major event
rate (p = 0.01)

Verapamil
Placebo

failure, the difference was significant. The 18-month overall mortality rate (7.7 per cent versus 11.8 per cent) and major events rate (14.6 per cent versus 19.7 per cent) were significantly reduced in the verapamil group compared with the placebo group (Figure 2.12). Long-term treatment with verapamil after an MI prevents reinfarction and death, with the most pronounced effects in patients without heart failure (DAVIT-II).

The more recently reported calcium antagonist reinfarction Italian study (CRIS) randomized 531 patients 7–21 days post-MI to 360 mg verapamil daily and 542 to placebo. The mean follow-up was 23.5 months. There was no difference in total mortality or cardiac mortality and the lower reinfarction rate on verapamil (39 versus 49) was not significant.[110]

Verapamil has not been investigated as extensively as the beta-blockers or the dihydropyridines. Its pharmacodynamic actions and the results of DAVIT-II (and some of those of DAVIT-I) suggest a long-term positive effect in secondary prevention.

☐ Diltiazem

Primary prevention
There are no clinical data to support the contention that diltiazem might prevent a first infarction.

Secondary prevention
Two trials have assessed the impact of diltiazem in MI patients and have shown benefit in the short term in those with non-Q-wave infarction and in the long term in those with good left ventricular function. Some regard these observations as providing good evidence that diltiazem has a useful cardioprotective role; others are sceptical about a drug that only seems to help a subgroup of the population at risk.

Acute study
The Multicentre Diltiazem Reinfarction Study[111] included 576 patients with non-Q-wave MI (which accounts for one-third of all MIs). They received diltiazem or placebo starting 24–72 h after the onset of symptoms and continuing for 14 days. The primary endpoint was reinfarction within 14 days. Secondary endpoints were post-MI angina and refractory angina. Recurrent MI was documented in 27 patients on placebo (9.3 per cent) and in 15 patients on diltiazem (5.2 per cent), which was significantly different. The 14-day mortality was similar but diltiazem reduced the frequency of refractory post-MI angina by 49.7 per cent.

Zannad et al[112] conducted a double-blind, placebo-controlled study in 34 patients within 6 h of the onset of MI. All patients received heparin and a constant infusion of lignocaine. The diltiazem-treated group showed a significant decrease of the infarction size, although the treated group was small.

Long-term study
The Multicenter Diltiazem Postinfarction Trial (MDPIT)[113] enrolled 2466 patients with MI. They received either diltiazem or placebo and were followed for 12–52 months (mean 25 months). The primary endpoints were total mortality and first cardiac event (cardiac death or non-fatal MI). There were 226 cardiac events in the placebo group and 202 in the diltiazem group (11 per cent reduction), which was not a statistically significant difference. There was no difference in total mortality rate. Diltiazem was associated with a significant reduction in the

incidence of the cardiac events in the 1909 patients (80 per cent) who did not have pulmonary congestion. But in 490 patients (20 per cent) with pulmonary congestion, diltiazem was associated with a significant increase of cardiac events.

In patients without pulmonary congestion, the cardiac event rates were 8 per cent for diltiazem and 11 per cent for placebo. In groups of patients with pulmonary congestion, cardiac event rates were 26 per cent for diltiazem and 18 per cent for placebo (Figure 2.13).

In the 68–80 per cent of patients with left ventricular ejection fraction greater than 40 per cent, diltiazem was associated with decreased incidence of cardiac death and cardiac events rate (6 per cent versus 10 per cent). However, in patients with left ventricular ejection fraction less than 40 per cent it was associated with a borderline statistically significant increase of cardiac death and cardiac events rate (26 per cent versus 20 per cent).

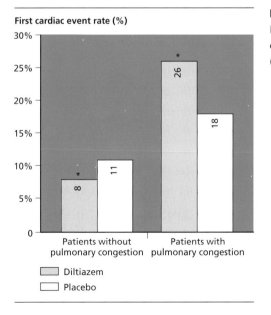

Figure 2.13
MDPIT, first cardiac event rate (p < 0.01).[113]

Although 55 per cent of patients were also taking beta-blockers, there were no significant interactions between these treatments.[113]

Subgroup analysis from the MDPIT study in 634 patients with non-Q-wave infarction during a follow-up of 1-year was performed. The cumulative 1-year cardiac event rate was 15 per cent in the placebo and 9 per cent in the diltiazem group. During the entire 52-month follow-up, there were 67 cardiac events in the placebo group and 41 in the diltiazem group, a significant 34 per cent reduction in event rate. There was an associated 30 per cent reduction in the total mortality and cumulative 38 per cent reduction in cardiac mortality. These results show that long-term prophylactic diltiazem treatment in patients with non-Q-wave MI is associated with a highly significant reduction in 1-year mortality.[114]

Diltiazem seems to help some post-MI patients; those who have a non-Q-wave infarction and those who do not develop pulmonary oedema. There are no primary prevention data. Further trials are needed to establish whether diltiazem could be considered a cardioprotective drug.

☐ Calcium antagonists – overall conclusions

The calcium antagonists are a group of drugs which have many actions suggesting that they might have an impact on CAD. Clinical trial data have so far provided little evidence to suggest that these drugs are cardioprotective. There is no evidence that any of the three groups of calcium antagonists will reduce the risk of having a first coronary event, and post-MI verapamil and diltiazem have only been shown to have an impact on patients with well-preserved cardiac function.

The possibility of an increased coronary mortality in those on short acting dihydropyridines[71–73] has raised concerns about this group of drugs. The evidence to date is that long-acting dihydropyridines[76] and other calcium antagonists do not have this adverse effect, though reservations about the group as a whole were expressed in the 1989 review by Held et al.[71] More recently, case control studies based on groups of elderly patients have suggested that calcium antagonists may increase the risk of gastrointestinal haemorrhage[115] and the risk of developing cancer.[116] The available data about cancer are conflicting. A later publication on a larger number of subjects using a validated information source[117] found a small positive association with cancer but concluded that because the risk did not increase with time it was not likely to be a causal association.[118]

■ ACE INHIBITORS

In the past decade the role of angiotensin-converting enzyme (ACE) inhibitors in the management of coronary heart disease (CHD) has extended enormously.[119–121] These drugs are no longer just of value in that minority of patients with severe heart failure at the end stage of the vicious cycle of CHD. Recent trials show that a much larger group of patients, at earlier stages in the vicious cycle, may now benefit from ACE inhibition (Figure 2.14).[119–121]

The following section reviews the broadening indications for ACE inhibitors in the light of the large clinical trials that have been reported since 1987 and the accompanying insights that these trials give into the mechanisms of action of ACE inhibitors.

□ Potential mechanisms of action of ACE inhibitors

Left ventricular dysfunction and heart failure

Activation of neural and endocrine reflexes is believed to be an integral component of the pathophysiology of the heart failure syndrome.[122] Teleologically, these reflexes are believed to be designed to restore tissue perfusion; from an evolutionary point of view, a situation of reduced tissue perfusion is most likely to arise as a consequence of haemorrhage rather than left ventricular dysfunction. Many of these reflexes, when activated, lead to arterial and venous vasoconstriction and sodium and water retention, i.e. hallmarks of the heart failure syndrome. Though appropriate in the situation of haemorrhage, these actions, by increasing preload and afterload, are believed to result in the failing heart failing further. Thus, neuroendocrine stimulation is believed to contribute to the progression of left ventricular dysfunction and

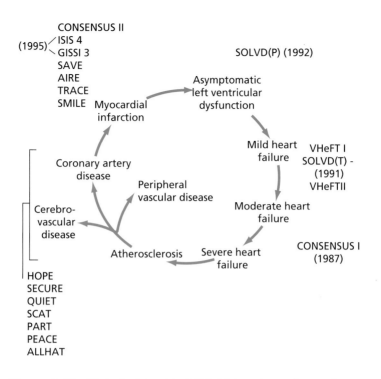

Figure 2.14 Clinical trials with ACE inhibitors in cardiovascular disease.

clinical deterioration (Figure 2.15).[122] The renin–angiotensin–aldosterone system (RAAS) is activated in overt heart failure and in asymptomatic left ventricular dysfunction,[123] and is further stimulated by diuretic therapy.[124] The RAAS not only has direct and disadvantageous vascular and renal actions, but also facilitates or stimulates other neural, endocrine and paracrine pathways with similarly adverse actions. These include arginine vasopressin and endothelin. The sympathetic nervous system is stimulated and the parasympathetic nervous system inhibited. These actions also lead to cardiac electrical instability, another hallmark of ventricular dysfunction. Angiotensin II, arginine

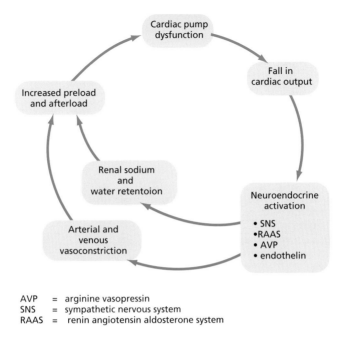

Cardiac pump
dysfunction

Fall in
cardiac output

Increased preload
and afterload

Neuroendocrine
activation

• SNS
•RAAS
• AVP
• endothelin

Renal sodium
and
water retentoin

Arterial and
venous
vasoconstriction

AVP   = arginine vasopressin
SNS   = sympathetic nervous system
RAAS =   renin angiotensin aldosterone system

Figure 2.15   Vicious cycle of heart failure.

vasopressin, endothelin and the sympathetic nervous system may, in addition, promote cardiac and vascular myocyte hypertrophy, leading to adverse structural change.[121,125] Angiotensin II and aldosterone may promote vascular and myocardial fibrosis which causes impaired muscle relaxation and further increases cardiac electrical instability. Finally, high circulating concentrations of angiotensin II are directly cardiotoxic, leading to myocyte necrosis.[126] By reducing the production of angiotensin II, ACE inhibitors attenuate or inhibit many of these direct and indirect hazardous actions of the RAAS in patients with left ventricular dysfunction. Comparative studies with other vasodilators, in which ACE inhibitors have emerged as more efficacious, have supported the 'neuroendocrine' hypothesis of heart failure.[127] Though often more powerful vasodilators than ACE inhibitors, and frequently leading to a greater improvement in left ventricular function, these other agents fail to lead to neuroendocrine suppression or may even cause neuroendocrine activation. New evidence in support of an adverse role of RAAS activation in the progression of heart failure comes from studies of the recently described ACE insertion/ deletion (ACE I/D polymorphism). Raynolds et al have found a greater prevalence of the DD genotype amongst patients with end-stage heart failure than in a normal control group.[128] This has been interpreted as indicating that the DD genotype, which is associated with increased blood and tissue ACE activity, predisposes to myocardial failure. The findings of Raynolds et al have, however, not been confirmed by others,[129] though another study has shown that patients with heart failure who are DD homozygotes have a worse prognosis.[130]

Left ventricular remodelling after myocardial infarction

Some years after it had been identified as a hallmark of heart failure, neuroendocrine activation was also shown to occur after MI. Neurohumoral stimulation is most pronounced in patients who develop acute cardiac failure at the time of infarction.[123] It also occurs, however, in a proportion of asymptomatic patients.[123] The greatest activation occurs in those with the greatest degree of left ventricular dysfunction. These patients are also those at highest risk of developing heart failure and premature death. It is likely that many of the actions of neuroendocrine stimulation believed to be harmful in heart failure are equally so in survivors of MI with left ventricular dysfunction. Local myocardial renin–angiotensin system activation may also be important in the pathophysiology of the progressive changes in the shape, size, wall thickness and function of the left ventricle that identify high-risk early survivors of MI, i.e. the changes that characterize progressive, decompensated, cardiac remodelling.[125] Increased expression of the messenger RNA for different components of the RAAS has been identified in both the infarction-related and infarction-remote areas of myocardium in such hearts.[131] Recent findings concerning the ACE I/D polymorphism have also suggested a key role for the RAAS in cardiac remodelling post-MI. Two small studies of MI survivors have found that DD homozygotes show increased left ventricular dilatation after infarction compared to those with the II genotype.[132,133] Another study, however, has shown no difference in survival after infarction according to the ACE genotype.[134]

Myocardial ischaemia and infarction

As reviewed below, there is recent intriguing but preliminary evidence that ACE inhibitors may also prevent recurrent coronary events in patients with left ventricular dysfunction. It should be emphasized that new coronary events are a further and underappreciated mechanism by which left ventricular dysfunction and heart failure progress (Figure 2.16). It is, therefore, somewhat artificial to separate the myocardial and coronary actions of ACE inhibitors.

It is also important to point out that, while ACE inhibitors may reduce *acute* coronary events, i.e. unstable angina and MI, they do not seem to have an anti-ischaemic action in chronic angina pectoris. Though perhaps surprising at first sight, there is some other evidence to suggest a role for the RAAS in acute coronary events. A large number of studies have investigated the relationship between the ACE I/D polymorphism and the risk of coronary events.[135] Though individually not all studies show such an association, collectively the evidence strongly supports an association between the D allele and MI.[135] Associations between CHD and polymorphisms for other components of the RAAS have also been identified.[136,137] In particular, the ACE I/D polymorphism and a polymorphism for the AT_1 receptor may interact to increase the risk of MI.[136]

Previously, plasma renin–sodium profile had also been shown to be an independent marker for increased risk of MI in patients

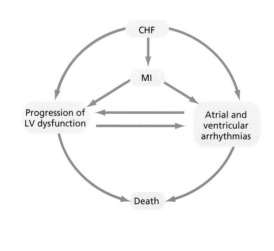

Figure 2.16 New coronary events and worsening heart failure.

with hypertension.[138] In this study, Alderman et al showed that the risk of MI was increased 5.3-fold amongst subjects with a higher versus those with a low renin profile. Interestingly, as in the ACE genotype studies, a high renin–sodium profile seemed to be particularly important in subjects otherwise at low risk, e.g. non-smokers and non-hyperlipidaemics. More recently, however, another study[139] has failed to confirm this association in *normotensive* individuals, though there was a trend for high renin to be associated with increased risk in men with higher blood pressures, in keeping with the findings of Alderman et al.[138]

Given that the acute ischaemic syndromes have two major pathophysiological components, i.e. plaque rupture and super-added thrombus formation, a number of theoretical mechanisms could explain the putative anti-ischaemic action of ACE inhibitors (Table 2.5). Whilst there is little clinical evidence for most of these effects, there are some important data from humans in support of a few of these putative actions.

Cardiac actions
- Restoring the balance between myocardial oxygen supply and demand
- Reduction in left ventricular preload and afterload
- Reduction in left ventricular mass
- Reduction in sympathetic stimulation

Vascular actions
- Direct antiatherogenic effect
- Antiproliferative and antimigratory effects on smooth muscle cells, neutrophils and mononuclear cells
- Improvement and/or restoration of endothelial function
- Protection from plaque rupture
- Antiplatelet effects
- Enhancement of endogenous fibrinolysis
- Antihypertensive effects
- Improvement in arterial compliance and tone

Table 2.5 Cardioprotective and vasculoprotective effects of angiotensin-converting enzyme inhibitors.

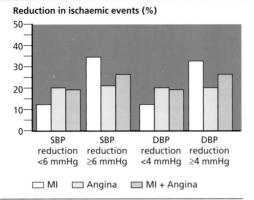

Figure 2.17 Effect of blood pressure reduction with enalapril on number of ischaemic events in SOLVD. SBP = systolic blood pressure, DBP = diastolic blood pressure; MI = myocardial infarction.

ACE inhibitors could influence plaque stability in a number of ways, not least by lowering blood pressure. In SAVE, a higher baseline systolic arterial pressure was associated with increased risk of reinfarction.[140] In SOLVD there was a trend for a greater reduction in blood pressure to be associated with a greater reduction in the risk of MI (Figure 2.17).[141]

ACE inhibitors may also reduce the risk of coronary thrombosis. There is evidence that angiotensin II stimulates the release of prothrombotic factors (e.g. plasminogen activator inhibitor, PAI-I) and inhibits the release of antithrombotic factors (e.g. tissue plasminogen activator, tPA) from the vascular endothelium, thus creating a clotting tendency.[142] ACE inhibitors seem to reverse this tendency.[143,144]

There is further evidence that ACE inhibitors may have an anticlotting action.

Tissue factor (TF) expression in monocytes and vascular smooth muscle cells is increased in patients with acute coronary syndromes and is capable of activating the clotting cascade in vivo by binding to essential cofactor VIII.[145] Treatment with an ACE inhibitor reduces the plasma concentration of TF antigen in patients after MI.[145] By reducing plasma adrenaline (epinephrine) concentrations, ACE inhibitors may also reduce platelet adhesiveness; indeed angiotensin II augments the aggregatory response of platelets to adrenaline.[146] Collectively, these

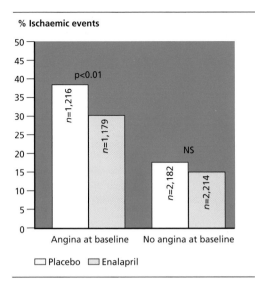

Figure 2.18
Effect of enalapril on MI or hospitalization for angina in SOLVD.

interesting observations suggest that, teleologically, the RAAS may be designed to maintain tissue perfusion not just by restoring blood volume and pressure but also by promoting blood coagulation. These responses would, of course, be highly appropriate if tissue perfusion was threatened by haemorrhage but very disadvantageous if tissue perfusion was reduced because of left ventricular dysfunction consequent upon CHD (Figure 2.18).

ACE inhibitors may also normalize coronary endothelial function in patients with CHD. A healthy endothelium appears to be a barrier to atherosclerosis as well as resisting platelet adhesion and thrombus formation. In the Trial on Reversing Endothelial Dysfunction (TREND) study, ACE inhibitor treatment was shown to improve the coronary vasodilator response to stimulated nitric oxide release in patients.[147] Whilst this may relate to the actions of ACE inhibition on the RAAS, it may also reflect the fact that kininase II, which is identical in structure to ACE, is also inhibited by these drugs. As a result, bradykinin degradation is inhibited and increased bradykinin concentrations in turn augment the local production of nitric oxide and vasodilatory prostaglandins in blood vessels.

	V-HeFT I			CONSENSUS I		SOLVD(T)		V-HeFT II	
	Placebo	Prazosin	H-ISDN	Placebo	Enalapril	Placebo	Enalapril	HISDN	Enalapril
n =	273	183	186	126	127	1284	1285	401	403
Mean age (years)	59	58	58	70	71	61	61	61	61
% male	100	100	100	71	70	80	81	100	100
NYHA II	–	–	–	0	0	57	57	52	50
III	–	–	–	0	0	31	30	42	44
IV	–	–	–	100	100	2	2	0.5	0.2
LVEF	30	29	30	–	–	25	25	29	29
IHD	44	44	44	74	72	72	70	52	54
Hypertension	43	40	40	19	24	42	43	45	50
Mean follow-up months		27.6		6.5		41.4		30.0	

n = subjects enrolled in each treatment group; H-ISDN = combination treatment with hydralazine and isosorbide dinitrate; NYHA = New York Heart Association classification; LVEF = left ventricular ejection fraction; IHD = ischaemic heart disease

Table 2.6 Breakdown of treatment groups in recent CHF studies.

☐ The heart failure trials

The major clinical trials in chronic heart failure are summarized in Table 2.6 and Figure 2.19.

Cooperative North Scandinavian Enalapril Survival Study (CONSENSUS I)

CONSENSUS I, published in 1987, was the first clinical trial to show that ACE inhibitors reduce mortality in chronic heart failure (CHF).[148] The patients randomized in CONSENSUS I had severe end-stage, mainly New York Heart Association (NYHA) Class IV, CHF. The relative and absolute reductions in mortality with enalapril were large (Figure 2.19).

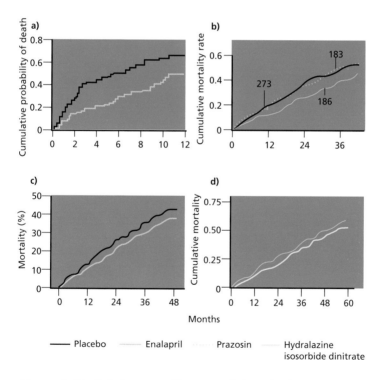

Figure 2.19 Relative mortaility rates of drugs in the major CHF studies. (a) CONSENSUS I; (b) V-HeFT I: (c) SOLVD (T); (d) V-HeFT II.

Several important features of this study should be noted.

First, the average age of patients was 70 years, the oldest of all the heart failure trials and an age typical of heart failure patients in clinical practice. The second point to note is that the patients randomized to CONSENSUS I were already treated with conventional therapy – 98 per cent were taking a loop diuretic, 93 per cent isosorbide dinitrate and 52 per cent spironolactone. The average dose of frusemide taken was 205 mg! The third important point about CONSENSUS I is that the target dose of enalapril was 20 mg twice daily, the largest target dose in any of the major clinical trials.

Perhaps the most important point to note from CONSENSUS I is the truly awful mortality in patients with advanced heart failure. The mortality in the placebo (conventional therapy) group exceeded 60 per cent at 1 year. Six-month mortality was reduced from 44 per cent to 26 per cent, a relative reduction of 31 per cent and an absolute reduction of 18 per cent. This reduction is equivalent to 160 fewer premature deaths per 1000 patient years of treatment, a clinical benefit unrivalled in any other trial. It should also be stressed that quality as well as quantity of life was improved by enalapril. After 6 months, 30 per cent of enalapril-treated and 20 per cent of placebo-treated patients had improved from NYHA Class IV to Class III CHF. Ten per cent of enalapril-treated patients had increased to Class II compared to 2 per cent of placebo-treated patients.

Interestingly, retrospective analyses of this trial, and some smaller ACE inhibitor trials, suggest that the major benefit was seen in those patients with CHF caused by underlying CAD (see below and Figure 2.20).

Studies of Left Ventricular Dysfunction (SOLVD) – treatment trial

In this much larger trial (Table 2.6), enalapril was shown to reduce mortality to a smaller extent in much less severely ill patients with mainly NYHA Class II and III CHF (Figure 2.19).[149]

In many ways the treatment arm of SOLVD is even more important than CONSENSUS I. The patients in SOLVD are in most respects (with the major exception of age) more representative of the majority of heart failure patients in the population, who tend to have mild to moderately severe symptoms rather than NYHA Class IV symptoms as in CONSENSUS I. By being much larger (more than 10 times as many patients) and by

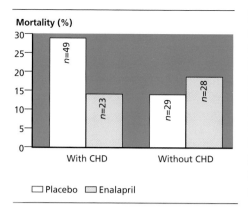

Figure 2.20 Effect of angiotensin converting enzyme (ACE) inhibition on martality in congestive heart failure patients in the Co-operative North Scandinavian Enalapril Survival Study (CONSENSUS I). CHD = coronary heart disease.

having a much longer follow-up (nearly seven times as long) than CONSENSUS I, SOLVD also gives a much more statistically robust estimate of the true benefits and hazards of ACE inhibitor therapy in CHF.

After 41.4 months of follow-up, placebo group mortality was 39.7 per cent and mortality in the enalapril group was 35.2 per cent, a relative risk reduction of 16 per cent ($P = 0.0036$) and an absolute reduction of 4 per cent. Though these percentages are much smaller than in CONSENSUS I, they will represent a large absolute benefit of 17 fewer deaths per 1000 patient years of treatment, a benefit larger than that obtained with many other therapies. In a public health sense, because the patients who went into SOLVD were more representative of the larger population of patients with heart failure, application of this clinical trial to clinical practice should have a much larger overall impact than CONSENSUS I.

SOLVD is also interesting because it emphasizes another benefit of ACE inhibitors. Enalapril reduced the need for hospitalization during the trial, particularly hospitalization for heart failure. In absolute terms, enalapril therapy resulted in 67 fewer hospitalizations for heart failure per 1000 patient years of treatment (and 100 fewer total hospitalizations per 1000 patient years). This effect probably reflects, amongst other things, the ability of ACE inhibitors to reduce the progression of heart failure from a mild to a severe stage.

Once again SOLVD confirmed that ACE inhibitors, in large doses, are well tolerated and bring about substantial reductions in morbidity and mortality.

Vasodilator–Heart Failure Trial II (V-HeFT II)

In this trial, there was a head-to-head comparison between enalapril and the vasodilator combination of hydralazine and ISDN (H-ISDN).[127] V-HeFT I had shown a reduction in mortality that was of borderline significance when H-ISDN was compared with placebo and prazosin, all three treatments being added to conventional therapy with diuretics and digoxin in patients with mainly NYHA Class II–III CHF (Figure 2.21).[150] In V-HeFT II, mortality was lower in the enalapril group than in the H-ISDN group.[127]

V-HeFT II merely confirmed the widespread clinical suspicions that hydralazine and ISDN, in combination, were both less well tolerated and less effective than ACE inhibitors in heart failure. Mortality was 28 per cent lower in Class II–III patients who received enalapril (32.8 per cent) than in those treated with H-ISDN (38.2 per cent), ($p = 0.016$ at 2 years of follow-up). Overall, enalapril treatment resulted in 22 fewer premature deaths per 1000 patient years of treatment compared to H-ISDN. This is a clinically substantial and meaningful advantage.

Though ACE inhibitors have undoubtedly been a huge advance in the treatment of heart failure, the prognosis of a patient who develops heart failure remains poor even with this treatment. For example, in the treatment arm of SOLVD, 35 per cent of patients with so-called 'mild' and 'moderate' heart failure, treated with enalapril, died within 3.5 years of follow-up. Forty-eight per cent died or were hospitalized for worsening heart failure and 59 per cent were hospitalized, at least once, for some reason during follow-up. Clearly, the most promising way to improve outcome in heart failure is to prevent its development. The natural history of most patients with heart failure is now clear. Its origins are in the coronary care unit at the time of MI. Patients may have signs of acute heart failure or be symptom-free immediately after infarction. A large proportion of apparently symptom-free patients have 'silent' left ventricular dysfunction and may go months or years before developing frank heart failure. The latest set of ACE inhibitor trials has looked at the possible role of these drugs in treating survivors of MI with a view to preventing the development of heart failure and premature death.

Asymptomatic left ventricular dysfunction

As it became established that ACE inhibitors were of benefit in all grades of symptomatic left ventricular dysfunction (i.e. CHF), clearly the next step was to evaluate the role of these drugs in patients with asymptomatic left ventricular dysfunction to see if progression to symptomatic heart failure could be prevented.

SOLVD – prevention trial

In the prevention trial of SOLVD, 4228 patients were randomized to either placebo or enalapril and followed up for approximately 4 years.[151] Eighty per cent of these patients had a history of MI. MI within the previous 30 days was an exclusion criterion in this trial, though 27 per cent of patients had had an MI between 30 days and 6 months before trial entry. Approximately one-third of patients reported angina at the time of randomization.

Though total mortality was not decreased by ACE inhibitor therapy, there was a significant reduction in the prespecified endpoints of development of CHF, hospitalization for CHF and the combination of these outcomes and death (Figure 2.6).

Enalapril treatment led to a 37 per cent reduction in the risk of developing heart failure, resulting in 30 fewer cases of heart failure per 1000 patient years of treatment. There were also 13 fewer first hospitalizations for heart failure per 1000 patient years of treatment in the enalapril group. These benefits were obtained over and above any benefit accruing from conventional therapy (24 per cent of enalapril-treated patients were receiving beta-blockers, 56 per cent antiplatelet therapy, 11 per cent anticoagulants and 30 per cent nitrates).

☐ Post-myocardial infarction trials

At the same time that the SOLVD prevention trial was being planned and initiated, other trials in patients with MI were getting underway. MI often leads to significant left ventricular damage and subsequent dilatation and dysfunction, both of which are frequently progressive. Patients who show progressive dysfunction have a poor prognosis with an increased risk of developing CHF and dying prematurely. Small, mechanistic studies had shown that early ACE inhibition in those high-risk patients could reduce left ventricular enlargement and, in experimental studies in animals, reduce mortality. It was hoped, therefore, that

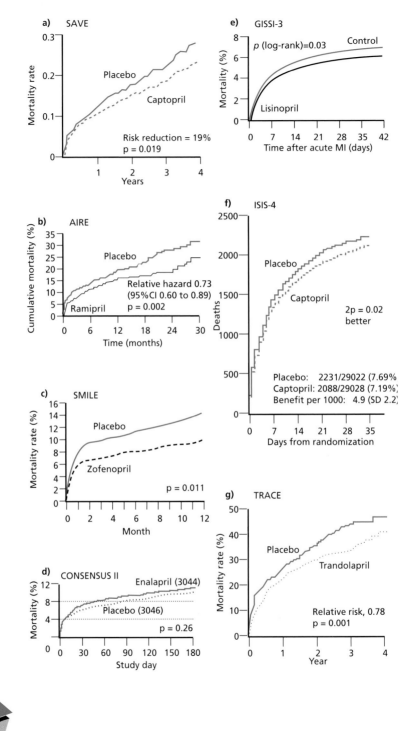

Figure 2.21 Event curves from the major trials of ACE inhibitor therapy after myocardial infarction: (a) Survival and Ventricular Enlargement study (SAVE); (b) Acute Infarction Rampiril Efficacy study (AIRE); (c) SMILE; (d) Co-operative North Scandinavian Enalapril Group (CONSENSUS II); (e) Third Gruppo Italiano per lo Studio Sopravvivenza nell-Infarto miocardico (GISSI-3); (f) Fourth International Study of Infarct Survival (ISIS-4); (g) Trandolapril Cardiac Evaluation (TRACE).

ACE inhibition might also reduce the risk of developing CHF and the risk of dying in patients with MI.

The post-MI trials are very heterogeneous but can, broadly, be divided into two groups (Figure 2.21, Table 2.7):

• those that selected higher-risk patients;
• those that were non-selective.

Selective trials

Chronologically, these were the Survival and Ventricular Enlargement study (SAVE),[140] Acute Infarction Ramipril Efficacy study (AIRE),[152] Survival of Myocardial Infarction Long-term Evaluation (SMILE)[153] and Trandolapril Cardiac Evaluation (TRACE).[154] The SAVE and TRACE trials selected patients on the basis of radionuclide ventriculographic or echocardiographic evidence of left ventricular dysfunction, respectively. AIRE selected patients on the basis of clinical and/or radiographic evidence of acute 'heart failure' (left ventricular failure). SMILE selected patients with an anterior Q-wave MI who had not received thrombolytic therapy, i.e. those patients most likely to have sustained significant left ventricular damage.[153]

Though there is some overlap between patients identified by the AIRE versus SAVE/TRACE/SMILE criteria, this is not complete. This is an important point, because:

Table 2.7 Post-infarction ACE inhibitor trials.

	SAVE	AIRE	TRACE	SMILE	CONSENSUS II	GISSI-3	ISIS-4
ACE-inhibitor initial dose	Captopril Test dose: 6.25 mg	Ramipril No test dose initially	Trandolapril Test dose: 0.5 mg	Zofenopril No test dose	Enalapril 1 mg enalaprilat iv over 2 hours	Lisinopril 5.0 mg	Captopril No test dose
Drug initiation after MI	3–16 days	3–10 days	3–7 days	<24 hours	<24 hours	<24 hours	<24 hours
Maintenance dose	Maximal tolerated up to 50 mg three times daily	Maximal tolerated up to 5 mg twice daily	Maximal tolerated up to 4 mg once daily	Maximal tolerated 30 mg twice daily	Maximal tolerated up to 20 mg once daily	Maximal tolerated up to 10 mg daily	Maximal tolerated 50 mg twice daily
Follow-up	2–5 years	6–30 months	2–4 years	6 weeks and 1 year	1.5–6 months	6 weeks and 6 months	5 weeks and 6 months
Post-MI population	EF ≤40% (radionuclide ventriculography)	Clinical evidence of heart failure (no EF)	WMI ≤1.2 (i.e. EF ≤35%) centralized echo	Anterior MI No thrombolysis	All (no EF)	All	All
Exclusions	Residual ischaemia overt heart failure	Severe heart failure, unstable angina	–	Congestive heart failure	–	Severe heart failure	Chronic use of high doses of diuretics
Proportion of screened patients randomized	6% (2231 out of 36 630 MIs)	6.5% (2006 out of 30 717 MIs)	25% (1749 out of 7010 MIs)	7.7%	59% (6090 out of 10 387 MIs)	45% (19 394 out of 43 047 MIs)	N/A
Overall 1-year mortality	~10%	~16%	24%	14%	–	–	–
Risk reduction	19%	27%	22%	29%†	No reduction observed	11%	7%*

AMI, acute myocardial infarction; EF, ejection fraction; WMI, wall motion index; †1 year; *5 weeks.

- there is a subgroup of patients who appear well clinically but are at significant risk of an adverse outcome;
- these asymptomatic patients gain a substantial benefit from ACE inhibitor treatment (Figure 2.21).

Non-selective trials

Chronologically, these trials were CONSENSUS II,[155] Gruppo Italiano per to Studio della Sopravvivenza nell-Infarcto miocardico (GISSI-3)[156] and the Fourth International Study of Infarct Survival (ISIS-4).[157,158] Essentially, these trials sought to randomize all patients without obvious contraindications (e.g. hypotension, renal impairment) to ACE inhibitor therapy. These trials, however, also differed in two further ways from the selective studies. First, treatment was started much earlier: within the first 24 h of admission in all three trials. Second, in two of the trials – GISSI-3 and ISIS-4 – treatment was given for a short period only, i.e. 4–6 h, after MI. In CONSENSUS II, treatment was also started via the intravenous route.[155]

Compared to the selective trials, only a very small ACE inhibitor benefit was seen in GISSI-3 and ISIS-4 (Figure 2.21) and no benefit was noted in CONSENSUS II. In GISSI-3 and ISIS-4 the benefit seemed to be confined to those with apparent or likely left ventricular dysfunction (Table 2.8).

	Proportion	35 day mortaility	Absolute mortality reduction with captopril
Heart failure	14%	14.7%	1.6%
Anterior and inferior MI	5%	9.0%	1.0%
Previous MI	17%	9.2%	1.7%
Anterior MI	34%	8.7%	1.3%

Table 2.8 ISIS-4 – Maximizing the benefit

☐ Trials in left ventricular dysfunction – conclusions

At the end of the first decade of the clinical story of ACE inhibitors, their indications have broadened dramatically from third-line therapy in severe end-stage CHF to first-line treatment for not only patients with any degree of CHF but also for those with, or at high risk of having, left ventricular dysfunction. This is because the totality of evidence from mechanistic and outcome studies shows that ACE inhibitors have clear clinical benefits in patients with left ventricular dysfunction irrespective of whether or not there are accompanying symptoms or signs of heart failure. The greatest absolute benefit, however, is seen in those with the greatest absolute risk, though the former constitute the minority of patients at risk.

☐ ACE inhibitors and coronary heart disease events

One of the surprising findings in the clinical trials of left ventricular dysfunction is the apparent beneficial effect of ACE inhibitors on CHD events, e.g. MI and unstable angina. This apparent effect has spawned a new set of major ACE inhibitor clinical outcome trials which will report in the second decade of the clinical history of these drugs (Table 2.9). Whereas the first generation of trials have established the role of ACE inhibitors in patients with left ventricular dysfunction, this second generation of trials will clarify whether ACE inhibitors have a much broader indication in the treatment of atherosclerotic disease, be it in the coronary, carotid or peripheral arteries.

Coronary heart disease events in SOLVD

In the combined arms of SOLVD, enalapril appeared to reduce the risk of developing an MI (or, more correctly, a recurrent MI) and unstable angina.[141] The event curves for both these outcomes did not, however, clearly separate until after 6–12 months (Figure 2.22).

Just over one-third of patients in both arms of SOLVD had symptoms of angina at baseline and these patients had the highest event rates and greatest benefit from enalapril.

Trial	ACE inhibitor	Primary outcome	Projected sample size	Duration of treatment
HOPE	Ramipril	Composite end point: cardiovascular death, myocardial infarction, and stroke	8000–9000	3.5 years
SECURE	Ramipril	B-mode ultrasound measures of carotid atherosclerosis	700	3.5 years
QUIET	Quinapril	A. Quantitative coronary angiographic measures of CAD progression B. Cardiac ischemic end points*	1775	3 years
SCAT	Enalapril	Quantitative coronary angiographic measures of CAD progression	468	5 years
PART	Ramipril	B-mode ultrasound measures of carotid atherosclerosis	600	4 years
PEACE	Trandolapril	Cardiovascular death/MI	14 000	3 years

ACE indicates angiotensin-converting enzyme; HOPE, Heart Outcomes Prevention Evaluation; SECURE, Study to Evaluate Carotid Ultrasound Changes with Ramipril and Vitamin E; QUIET, The Quinapril Ischemic Event Trial; SCAT, Simvastatin and Enalapril Coronary Atherosclerosis Trial; PART, Prevention of Atherosclerosis with Ramipril Therapy; and CAD, coronary artery disease.
*Composite end point including cardiovascular death, nonfatal myocardial infarction, coronary revascularization procedures (coronary artery bypass graft surgery, angioplasty, atherectomy), and hospitalization for unstable angina pectoris.

Table 2.9 Summary of major ongoing long-term trials examining the effects of ACE inhibitors on atherosclerotic disease progression or ischemic events in patients without heart failure or low ejection fraction

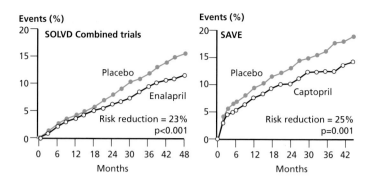

Figure 2.22 Incidence of myocardial infarction in the SOLVD prevention trial and incidence of recurrent myocardial infarction in the SAVE trial.

Though fewer patients had a history of MI in the treatment arm of SOLVD (66 per cent versus 80 per cent in the prevention arm), there was a higher cumulative incidence of unstable angina in the treatment arm of SOLVD (18.7 per cent versus 16.8 per cent, treatment arm versus prevention arm).

In SOLVD, as in SAVE and AIRE (see below), interim MI had a grave effect on prognosis. One-year mortality was 55 per cent amongst the patients (650 patients) who had had MI compared to 7 per cent amongst those who did not. One-quarter of all deaths in SOLVD were preceded by an interim MI. One-third of deaths were preceded by interim MI or admission to hospital with unstable angina.

Coronary heart disease events in SAVE

Though captopril did not reduce the incidence of unstable angina in SAVE, there was an apparent 25 per cent reduction in the rate of recurrent MI with active therapy, i.e. a proportional reduction similar to that reported in SOLVD (Figure 2.9).[140] In SAVE, however, there has been some controversy about the definition of recurrent MI. Despite this, and as in SOLVD, recurrent MI had important prognostic implications, increasing the risk of death seven-fold (the increased risk in SOLVD was 7.8-fold). In SAVE, recurrent MI increased the risk of developing severe CHF three-fold (33 per cent versus 11 per cent, in patients not having recurrent MI).

In contrast to SOLVD, ACE inhibitor treatment did not reduce the need for hospitalization for unstable angina in SAVE.

Interestingly, however, captopril reduced the need for revascularization (by surgery or angioplasty) in the SAVE trial by about a quarter. This surprising finding is in keeping with other recent reports that captopril may prevent or reduce reversible myocardial ischaemia post-MI (see below).

☐ Coronary heart disease events in other major post-MI trials

Active treatment with an ACE inhibitor had no effect on the risk of recurrent MI in CONSENSUS II,[155] GISSI-3[156] or ISIS-4.[157] These trials may not, however, have been able to detect an effect of ACE inhibition on the risk of MI because their duration of treatment and follow-up was so short.

TRACE[154] has not yet reported on the risk of MI.

In AIRE,[152] there was a trend for a reduced risk of myocardial reinfarction with ramipril, though the number of patients randomized and relatively short follow-up meant that the study was probably unable to answer this question reliably. As in SOLVD and SAVE, interim MI had an adverse prognostic impact in AIRE.

In TRACE there was a strong trend to a reduction in recurrent MI.

☐ Coronary heart disease events in other large ACE inhibitor trials

Two other large trials are also of interest with respect to the question of whether ACE inhibitors have an effect on CHD events.[152,153]

The Multicenter American Research Trial with Cilazapril after Angioplasty to Prevent Transluminal Coronary Obstruction (MARCATOR)[158] and the Multicenter European Research Trial with Cilazapril after Angioplasty to Prevent Transluminal Coronary Obstruction (MERCATOR)[159] are trials in which patients undergoing coronary angioplasty were randomized to placebo or the ACE inhibitor cilazapril. The purpose of the trials was to determine whether or not ACE inhibitor therapy would reduce the risk of coronary restenosis following angioplasty. Cilazapril did not reduce the risk of restenosis and had no effect on the rate of CHD events in either trial.

☐ Quinapril ischaemic event trial (QUIET)

QUIET was a randomized placebo-controlled trial designed to study the effect of quinapril on ischaemic events (cardiac death, non-fatal MI, resuscitated ventricular arrhythmias, revascularization procedures and hospital admissions for angina) during the long-term follow-up of 1750 patients who had undergone coronary angioplasty.[160,161] The preliminary results of this study were presented at the meeting of the European Society of Cardiology in Birmingham, August 1996. The number of endpoints in the quinapril group was similar to that in the placebo group, i.e. there was no evidence that quinapril reduced the incidence of ischaemic events. The number of 'hard events' (i.e. death, MI, significant ventricular arrhythmias) was, however, very small (57 placebo, 48 quinapril, hazard ratio 0.87, 0.59–1.29), and this trial was probably underpowered in terms of showing, definitively, whether or not ACE inhibitors really do have an effect on acute coronary events. The results of larger trials are, therefore, still eagerly awaited.

☐ Summary and conclusions – looking to the future

There is no doubt that treatment for all patients with ACE inhibitors is indicated where there is left ventricular dysfunction. Treatment for all patients with CAD is not yet indicated. The SOLVD and SAVE studies have provided intriguing data to suggest that ACE inhibitors may prevent CHD events, but these early observations require confirmation. In this respect, several large trials are already planned (or underway) and will begin to report in the next five years (Table 2.9).

■ ALPHA-ADRENERGIC BLOCKING DRUGS

The selective postjunctional alpha$_1$ adrenergic blocking drugs (alpha-blockers) such as prazosin, doxazosin and terazosin represent a striking improvement as antihypertensive agents compared with earlier alpha-blockers. These drugs have the potential to modify several risk factors for cardiovascular disease.

Effects of plasma lipid profile

The level of cholesterol and especially the total cholesterol/(HDL) cholesterol ratio are considered important CHD risk factors.[162] Several studies have demonstrated a favourable effect of alpha$_1$-blocker therapy on lipid metabolism;[163–165] whereas other antihypertensive drugs adversely affect plasma lipids or are 'lipid-neutral'.

Prazosin produces a fall in total triglycerides, total cholesterol, LDL cholesterol and VLDL cholesterol, and causes an increase in HDL cholesterol concentration of 2–15 per cent.[166–169] Doxazosin and terazosin have similar effects.[170–172] Doxazosin has favourable effects on lipid profiles in patients with type II diabetes mellitus and hypertension.[171–173]

A meta-analysis of the pooled data from several studies, including 5413 hypertensive patients on doxazosin, has shown significant reduction of LDL cholesterol by 4.8 per cent and of triglycerides by 7.6 per cent, and significant increase of the total cholesterol/HDL cholesterol ratio by 5.8 per cent[174] (Figure 2.23).

Alpha-blockers also stimulate lipoprotein lipase and lecithin cholesterol acyltransferase (LCAT) activity,[175] which may be responsible for triglyceride reduction and the HDL cholesterol increase. Leren[176] found that doxazosin stimulates LDL receptors in fibroblasts, suggesting enhanced catabolism of LDL. Alpha-blockers may also modify the adrenergic regulation of cholesterol synthesis.[177]

Effects on insulin sensitivity

Insulin resistance is often associated with hypertension and type II diabetes and may lead to sodium retention and disturbances in glucose and lipid metabolism, which all increase the risk for CHD.

Alpha-blockers have been shown to improve insulin sensitivity in hypertensive patients with impaired glucose tolerance and

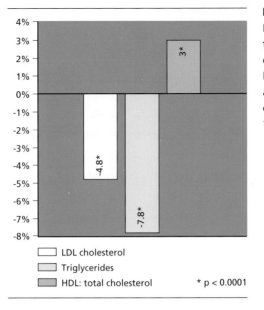

Figure 2.23
Pooled data on the effects of doxazosin on the LDL, triglycerides, and HDL/total cholesterol ratio.[174] *$p < 0.05$.

☐ LDL cholesterol
☐ Triglycerides
☐ HDL: total cholesterol   * $p < 0.0001$

insulin resistance.[178] Prazosin significantly improved insulin-mediated glucose disposal in moderately obese hypertensive patients.[179] Furthermore, doxazosin has been shown to reduce serum levels of insulin and glucose in hypertensive patients.[172,180] These changes in blood glucose levels and serum insulin sensitivity in hypertensive patients could favourably affect the probability of developing CHD. Alpha-blockers have no impact on serum potassium or uric acid concentrations.[165]

Effects on ventricular hypertrophy

Hypertension is the main cause of left ventricular hypertrophy, which has been shown to be an important independent risk factor for CHD. In hypertensive patients, treatment with prazosin,[181] doxazosin,[182] and terazosin[183] significantly reduced left ventricular mass. This reduction is probably due to reduction in left ventricular wall stress as a result of decreased peripheral vascular resistance.

Antithrombotic effects of alpha-blockers

In hypertensive patients, induced platelet aggregation is significantly reduced by doxazosin compared with placebo.[184] In 84 hypertensive patients, doxazosin improved the activity of the fibrinolytic system (TPA increased significantly).[185]

☐ Primary prevention

Long-term comparative studies involving large populations have confirmed that monotherapy with prazosin, doxazosin and terazosin[167,168,172,186] produces a significant and sustained reduction in blood pressure in patients with mild-to-moderate hypertension. However, despite their beneficial effects on some risk factors, there is no good evidence that alpha-blockers have produced a reduction in CHD morbidity and mortality, since the appropriate studies have not yet been done. A possible benefit of alpha-blockers in preventing CHD will only be determined after obtaining the results of long-term comparison studies of alpha-blockers with CHD morbidity and mortality as endpoints. The Treatment of Mild Hypertension (TOHMS) Study did not address the subject adequately.[187]

There is a large database on use of alpha-blockers in patients with heart failure. Furberg and Yusuf[188] reviewed nine trials with alpha-blockers in heart failure and concluded that they probably do not improve survival.

☐ Secondary prevention

Alpha-blockers are not used in post-MI patients.

■ ORGANIC NITRATES

Nitrates have been used for over 100 years to relieve the pain of angina pectoris.[189] More recently, efforts have been directed to finding an effective long acting preparation that could be used prophylactically and which is not rendered ineffective because of the development of tolerance.[190,191] In addition, intravenous nitrates are now being used extensively in the management of patients with AMI and those with acute left ventricular failure. Not only do they relieve symptoms, but early studies suggested that they also reduce coronary mortality.[192]

The increasing use of nitrates has been associated with and possibly, in part, caused by, advances in our understanding of the many ways in which these drugs might influence CAD. A nitrate preparation was included in the ISIS-4 study,[157] as the evidence suggested a role for nitrates as potential cardioprotective drugs.

☐ Mechanisms

The basic haemodynamic effects of nitrates are well known. However, the large number of detailed investigations performed in recent years have added greatly to our understanding of these. Nitrates are predominantly vasodilators that reduce venous return, pulmonary oedema and heart work.[193] They also dilate peripheral arteries and lower peripheral resistance, which also reduces heart work.[194] In addition, they dilate coronary arteries, improve collateral flow, open up regions of stenotic narrowing and relax vasospasm.[195] Nitrates influence several processes that contribute to the morbidity and mortality from CAD.

Impact on diseased vessels

Endothelium-derived relaxing factor (EDRF) acts as a vasodilator in normal vessels. The active constituent is believed to be nitric oxide or a closely related substance. When the endothelium is damaged by atheromatous disease[196] or even by hypercholesterolaemia, vasodilatation may be impaired. Organic nitrates, such as those used therapeutically, are converted in the vessel wall by various steps that include a reaction with sulphydryl groups to form nitric oxide and are thus able to act as an 'exogenous EDRF'. Furthermore, when the endothelium is damaged, nitrates seem to be more effective vasodilators,[195] making them potentially valuable therapeutic agents in patients with acute or chronic myocardial ischaemia due to endothelial disease.

Modification of platelet function

The role of nitrates as antiaggregatory agents that tend to modify platelet function and reduce the risk of clotting has been demonstrated in several studies[197-199] but remains a subject of debate.[195] Platelets play a key part in clot formation, often the final step in the development of a coronary occlusion. Enhanced platelet activity has been documented in patients with AMI or unstable angina,[200] and this activity tends to increase during the early hours of the day, when MIs and episodes of silent ischaemia are most likely to occur.[201]

Left ventricular remodelling

Remodelling after MI leads to wall thinning, cavity dilatation and impaired function. Left ventricular end-systolic volume is a predictor of mortality, and patients who develop large left ventricles are more prone to cardiac failure, left ventricular aneurysms and risk of death from cardiac disease. In animals and in humans, nitrates and ACE inhibitors have been shown to suppress this deleterious remodelling process.[202,203]

Anti-ischaemic effects

Early studies at the Johns Hopkins University Hospital evaluated the haemodynamic effects of intravenous nitroglycerin in patients with an AMI.[204] Not only did the treatment improve left ventricular function, but it also reduced ischaemic damage as assessed by ST segment mapping.

Several other studies have demonstrated that infarction size may be reduced by intravenous nitroglycerin given early after the onset of symptoms of MI. Bussman et al[205] compared 31 treated patients with 29 control patients and showed an overall 23 per cent reduction in infarction size as determined by plasma creatine kinase concentrations. Jaffe et al[206] also showed a reduction in CK infarction size but only in patients with inferior infarctions. Derrida et al[207] showed a beneficial impact on ECG changes, and Jugdutt and Warnica[202] again showed a decrease in CK infarction size and 3-month mortality. The effects on CK infarction size are shown in Figures 2.24 and 2.25.

The reduction in infarction size found in these studies may in part be explained by the fact that nitrates tend to improve collateral flow both in animal models[208] and in humans.[209]

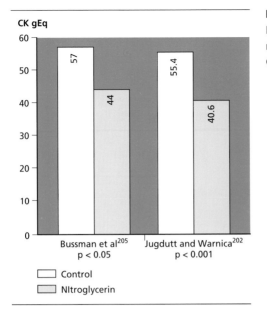

Figure 2.24
Impact of nitroglycerin on CK infarction size.

CK gEq

- Bussman et al[205] p < 0.05
- Jugdutt and Warnica[202] p < 0.001

☐ Control
▨ NItroglycerin

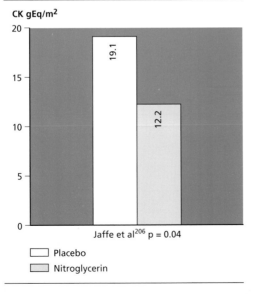

Figure 2.25
Impact of nitroglycerin on CK infarction size after inferior MI.

CK gEq/m^2

Jaffe et al[206] p = 0.04

☐ Placebo
▨ Nitroglycerin

☐ Primary prevention

There are no data to show that nitrates have a role in primary prevention.

☐ Secondary prevention

In 1988, Yusuf et al[192] completed a meta-analysis of 10 trials of nitrate therapy (three nitroprusside, seven nitroglycerin). Most of these trials contained relatively small numbers of patients, but all involved the administration of intravenous therapy started soon after the onset of symptoms associated with MI and continued for 48–72 h. The overall result for nitroprusside was a non-significant reduction in mortality (17.8 per cent on placebo, 14.3 per cent on active therapy). Intravenous nitroglycerin produced a significant reduction in mortality (20.5 per cent on placebo, 12.0 per cent on active treatment).

In March 1995, the report on ISIS-4 was published in *The Lancet*.[157] In this major study, the impact of 4 weeks of treatment with captopril and oral controlled-release mononitrate, and 24 h of intravenous magnesium sulphate, were documented; 58 050 patients were entered within 24 h of an acute MI into a $2 \times 2 \times 2$ factorial design study. Thus for each treatment there were about 29 000 treated patients and 29 000 controls. During the first 5 weeks there were 2129 (7.34 per cent) deaths among 29 018 mononitrate patients compared with 2190 (7.54 per cent) among 29 032 controls – a non-significant 3 per cent reduction in the risk of death. The paper also reviews the other trials and gives the overall data from the major trials for which results had been reported before March 1995. Overall, there had been 3012/40 974 (7.35 per cent) deaths on nitrates and 3166/40 934 (7.73 per cent) in the controls. Two important conclusions can be drawn. First, nitrates do not reduce coronary mortality in the early post-MI period, and nor do they cause serious adverse effects. A second useful observation was that headache, the major adverse effect of nitrate therapy, occurred in 3.21 per cent on nitrates and in 0.44 per cent of the controls.

Until recently, nitrates were considered to be simple vasodilators, undoubtedly effective in the management of acute angina, but one of the least exciting groups of cardiovascular drugs. They are now seen to have several cardioprotective effects in addition to their valuable haemodynamic actions. The results of ISIS-4[157] GISSI 3[156] and the other studies indicate that nitrates do not reduce mortality but they have few adverse effects and virtually no contraindications. They will continue to be used for their haemodynamic benefits.

■ CONCLUSION

Several different classes of drugs used to treat patients with hypertension and angina or those who have had an infarction have been discussed. No single preparation can be claimed to be the most effective, the best tolerated, the easiest to use and the most likely to prevent cardiovascular complications. Furthermore, the requirements of patients differ and the presence of other disease and the taking of other medication will influence the choice of antihypertensive and antianginal agent. However, since major coronary events and sudden death are the most common complications of hypertension, angina and the post-MI state, one should be aware of the potential of the preparations to reduce the patient's risk of developing these complications. All the drugs described have *some* capacity to reduce *some* risk factors and so should have *some* impact on the underlying disease. To date, only for beta-blockers can a claim be made that they have an impact on several of the pathological processes that lead to death from CAD. In addition, there are some primary prevention data in males and convincing secondary prevention data. ACE inhibitors have several potentially beneficial effects on CAD and they seem to reduce the risk of MI in patients with heart failure and in post-MI patients followed for long enough. Clinical data are limited for verapamil and diltiazem and are lacking for nitrates, dihydropyridines and alpha-blockers.

In patients known to have hypertension or CAD, not only should appropriate treatment be offered as indicated above, but also the risks from hyperlipidaemia, thromboembolism, arrhythmias and being post-menopausal should be considered. Deaths from a multifunctional disease are unlikely to be strikingly reduced by attempting to modify one risk factor alone.

References

1. MRC Working Party, Medical Research Council trial of treatment of hypertension in older adults: principal results, *Br Med J* (1992) **304**:405–12.

2. SHEP Cooperative Research Group, Prevention of stroke by antihypertensive drug treatment in dlder persons with isolated systolic hypertension, *JAMA* (1991) **265**:3255–64.

3. Dahlof B, Lindholm LH, Hansson L et al, Morbidity and mortality in the Swedish Trial in old patients with hypertension (STOP-Hypertension), *Lancet* (1991) **338**:1281–5.

4. Siegel D, Hulley SB, Black DM et al, Diuretics, serum and intracellular electrolytes levels, and ventricular arrhythmias in hypertensive men, *JAMA* (1992) **267**:1083–9.

5. Bigger JT, Diuretic therapy, hypertension and cardiac arrest, *N Engl J Med* (1994) **330**:1899–900.

6. Veterans Administration Cooperative Study Group on Antihypertensive Agents, Effects of treatment on morbidity in hypertension II. Results of patients with diastolic blood pressure averaging 90 through 114 mmHg, *JAMA* (1970) **213**:1143–51.

7. Australian National Blood Pressure Study Management Committee, The Australian therapeutic trial in mild hypertension, *Lancet* (1980) **i**:1261–7.

8. MacMahon SW, Cutler JA, Furberg CD and Payne GH. The effects of drug treatment for hypertension: a review of randomised clinical trials, *Prog Cardiovasc Dis* (1986) **29** (suppl 1):99–118.

9. Collins R, Peto R, McMahon S et al, Blood pressure, strokes and coronary heart disease. Part 2, short term reductions in blood pressure: overview of randomised drug trials in their epidemiological context, *Lancet* (1990) **335**:827–38.

10. Medical Research Council Working Party, MRC trial of treatment of mild hypertension: principal results, *Br Med J* (1985) **59**:364–78.

11. Wikstrand J, Warnold I, Olsson G, Toumilehto J, Elmfeldt D, Berglund G, on behalf of the Advisory Committee, Primary prevention with metoprolol in patients with hypertension. Mortality results from the MAPHY study, *JAMA* (1988) **259**:1976–82.

12. Wikstrand J, Warnold I, Tuomilehto J, Olsson G, Elmfeldt D, Berglund G, on behalf of the Advisory Committee, Metoprolol versus thiazide diuretics in hypertension. Morbidity results from the MAPHY study, *Hypertension* (1991) **17**:579–88.

13. Multiple Risk Factor Intervention Trial Research Group, Multiple Risk Factor Intervention Trial: risk factor changes and mortality results, *JAMA* (1982) **248**:1465–77.

14. Siscovick DS, Raghunathan TE, Psaty BM et al. Diuretics therapy for hypertension and the risk of primary cardiac arrest, *N Engl J Med* (1994) **330**:1852–7.

15. Hoes AW, Grobbee DF, Lubsen J et al, Diuretics, beta-blockers, and the risk of sudden cardiac death in hypertensive patients, *Ann Intern Med* (1995) **123**:481–7.

16. Pooling Project Research Group, Relationship of blood pressure, serum cholesterol, smoking habit, relative weight and ECG abnormalities to incidence of major coronary events. Final report of the Pooling Project, *J Chronic Dis* (1978) **31**:201–306.

17. Holme I, Enger SC, Helgeland A et al, Risk factors and raised atherosclerotic lesions in coronary and cerebral arteries. Statistical analysis from the Oslo study, *Atherosclerosis* (1981) **1**:250–6.

18. Kannel WB, Thomas HE, Sudden coronary death. The Framingham Study, *Ann NY Acad Sci* (1982) Part 1: 3–20.

19. Disdale JE, A perspective on type A behaviour and coronary disease, *N Engl J Med* (1988) **318**:110–12.

20. Pettersson K, Benjne B, Bjork H, Strawn WB, Bondjers G, Experimental sympathetic activation causes endothelial injury in the rabbit thoracic aorta via B-adrenoceptor activation, *Circ Res* (1990) **67**:1027–34.

21. Zarins CK, Giddens DP, Bharadray BK, Sottiurai VS, Mabon RF, Glagov S, Carotid bifurcation atherosclerosis. Quantitative correlation of plaque localisation with flow velocity profiles and wall shear stress, *Circ Res* (1983) **53**:502–14.

22. Thubrikar MJ, Christie AM, Cao-Danh HC, Holloway PE, Nolan SP, Metoprolol reduces low density lipoprotein uptake in aortic regions prone to atherosclerosis, *FASEB J* (1990) **4**:A1151.

23. Kaplan JR, Manuck SB, Adams MR et al, Propranolol inhibits coronary atherosclerosis in behaviourally predisposed monkeys fed an atherogenic diet, *Circulation* (1987) **76**:1364–72.

24. Strawn W, Bondjers G, Kaplan JR et al, Endothelial dysfunction response to psychosocial stress in monkeys, *Circ Res* (1991) **68**:1270–9.

25. Spence JD, Perkins DG, Klein RL, Adams MR, Haust MD, Hemodynamic modifications of aortic atherosclerosis: effects of propranolol versus hydralazine in hypertensive hyperlipidemic rabbits, *Atherosclerosis* (1984) **50**:325–33.

26. Kaplan JR, Manuck SB, Adams MR, Clarkson TB, The effects of beta-adrenergic blocking agents on atherosclerosis and its complications, *Eur Heart J* (1987) **8**:928–44.

27. Oslund-Lindqvist AM, Lindquist P, Brautigam J, Olsson G, Bondjers G, Nordborg C, The effect of metoprolol on diet-induced atherosclerosis in rabbits, *Atherosclerosis* (1988) **8**:40–4.

28. Linden T, Camejo G, Wiklund O, Warnold I, Olofsson S-O, Bondjers G, Effect of short-term beta blockade on serum lipid levels and on the interaction of LDL with human arterial proteoglycans, *J Clin Pharmacol* (1990) **30**: S123–31.

29. Fitzgerald JD, By what means might beta-blockers prolong life after acute myocardial infarction? *Eur Heart J* (1987) **8**:945–51.

30. Frishman WH, Christodouou J, Weksler B, Smithen C, Killip T, Scheidt S, Abrupt propranolol withdrawal in angina pectoris: effects on platelet aggregation and exercise tolerance, *Am Heart J* (1978) **95**:169–79.

31. Willich SN, Pohjola-Sintonen S, Bhatia SHS et al, Suppression of silent ischaemia by metoprolol without alteration of morning increase of platelet aggregability in patients with stable coronary artery disease, *Circulation* (1989) **79**:557–65.

32. Ablad B, Bjorkman JA, Gustafsson-D et al, The role of sympathetic activity in atherogenesis: effects of B-blockade, *Am Heart J* (1988) **116**:322–7.

33. Winther K, The effect of beta blockade on platelet function and fibrinolytic function, *J Cardiovasc Pharmacol* (1987) **10** (suppl 2):S94–8.

34. Roberts R, Modification of infarct size, *Circulation* (1980) **61**:458–9.

35. Leading Article. Long-term and short-term beta blockade after myocardial infarction, *Lancet* (1982) **i**: 1159–61.

36. Hjalmarson A, Elmfledt D, Herlitz J et al, Effect on mortality of metoprolol in acute myocardial infarction, *Lancet* (1981) **ii**: 823–7.

37. Peter T, Norris RM, Clarke ED et al, Reduction of enzyme levels by propranolol after acute myocardial infarction, *Circulation* (1978) **57**:1091–5.

38. Yusuf S, Ramsdale D, Peto R, Bennett D, Furse C, Sleight P, Early intravenous atenolol treatment in suspected acute myocardial infarction. Preliminary report of a randomised trial, *Lancet* (1980) **ii**: 273–6.

39. Skinner JE, Regulation of cardiac vulnerability by the cerebral defense system, *J Am Coll Cardiol* (1985) **5**:88B-94B.

40. Parker GW, Michael LH, Hartley CH, Skinner JE, Entman ML, Central B-adrenergic mechanisms may modulate ischaemic ventricular fibrillation in pigs, *Circ Res* (1990) **66**:259–70.

41. Dellsperger KC, Martins JB, Clothier JL, Marcus ML: Incidence of sudden cardiac death associated with coronary artery occlusion in dogs with hypertension and left ventricular hypertrophy is reduced by chronic B-adrenergic blockade, *Circulation* (1990) **82**: 941–50.

42. Ablad B, Bjuro T, Bjorkman JA, Edstrom T, Olsson G, Role of central nervous beta-adrenoceptors in the prevention of ventricular fibrillation through augmentation of cardiac vagal tone, *J Am Coll Cardiol* (1991) **17**:165A.

43. Olsson G, Tuomilehto J, Berglund G et al, Primary prevention of sudden cardiovascular death in hypertensive patients: mortality results from the MAPHY study, *Am J Hypertens* (1991) **4**:151–8.

44. Norwegian Study Group, Timolol-induced reduction in mortality and reinfarction in patients surviving acute myocardial infarction, *N Engl J Med* (1981) **304**:801–7.

45. Beta Blocker Heart Attack Trial Research Group, A randomized trial of propranolol in patients with acute myocardial infarction. 1. Mortality results, *JAMA* (1982) **247**:1707–13.

46. Ryden L, Ariniego R, Arnman K et al, A double-blind trial of metoprolol in acute myocardial infarction. Effect on ventricular arrhythmias, *N Engl J Med* (1983) **308**:614–18.

47. Murray DS, Murray RG, Littler WA, The effects of metoprolol given early in acute myocardial infarction on ventricular arrhythmias, *Eur Heart J* (1986) **7**:217–22.

48. Green KG, British MRC trial of treatment for mild hypertension – a more favourable interpretation, *Am J Hypertens* (1991) **4**:723–4.

49. The IPPPSH Collaborative Group, Cardiovascular risk and risk factors in a randomized trial of treatment based on the beta-blocker oxprenolol: The International Prospective Primary Prevention Study in Hypertension (IPPPSH), *J Hypertens* (1985) **3**:379–92.

50. Wilhelmsen L, Berglund G, Elmfeldt D et al, Beta-blockers versus diuretics in hypertensive men: main results from the HAPPHY trial, *J Hypertens* (1987) **5**:561–72.

51. Holme I, MAPHY and the two arms of HAPPHY, *JAMA* (1989) **262**:3272–4.

52. Kaplan NM, Critical comments on recent literature: SCRAAPHY about MAPHY from HAPPHY, *Am J Hypertens* (1988) **1**:428–30.

53. Moser M, Sheps S, Confusing messages from the newest of the beta-blockers/diuretics hypertension trials, *Arch Intern Med* (1989) **149**: 2174–5.

54. Wikstrand J, Primary prevention in patients with hypertension: comments on the clinical implications of the MAPHY trial, *Am Heart J* (1988) **116**: 338–47.

55. Wikstrand J, Kendall MJ, The role of beta-blockers in preventing sudden death, *Eur Heart J* (1992) **13** (suppl D):111–20.

56. Coope J, Warrender TS, Randomised trial of treatment of hypertension in elderly patients in primary care, *Br Med J* (1986) **293**: 1145–51.

57. Held P, Yusuf S, Early intravenous beta blockade in acute myocardial infarction, *Cardiology* (1989) **76**:132–43.

58. ISIS-1 (First international Study of Infarct Survival) Collaborative Group, Mechanisms for the early mortality reduction by beta-blockade started early in acute myocardial infarction, ISIS-1, *Lancet* (1988) **I**:921-3.

59. The MIAMI trial Research Group, Metoprolol in acute myocardial infarction (MIAMI), A randomised placebo-controlled international trial, *Eur Heart J* (1985) **6**:199–226.

60. Olsson G, Wikstrand J, Warnold I et al, Metoprolol induced reduction in post-infarction mortality: pooled results from five double-blind randomized trials, *Eur Heart J* (1992) **13**:28–32.

61. Kennedy HL, Rosenson RS, Physician use of beta-adrenergic blocking therapy: a changing perspective, *J Am Coll Cardiol* (1995) **26**:547–52.

62. Lau J, Antman EM, Jimenz-Silva J, Kupelnick B, Mosteller F, Chalmers TC, Cumulative meta-analysis of therapeutic trials for myocardial infarction, *N Engl J Med* (1992) **327**:248–54.

63. Soumerai SB, McLaughlin TJ, Spiegelman D et al, Adverse outcomes of underuse of beta-blockers in elderly survivors of acute myocardial infarction, *JAMA* (1997) **277** (2):115–21.

64. Kendall MJ, Lynch KP, Hjalmarson A, Kjekshus J, Beta blockers and sudden cardiac death, *Ann Intern Med* (1995) **123**:358–67.

65. Ayanian J, Hauptman PJ, Guadagnoli E et al, Knowledge and practices of generalist and specialist physicians regarding drug therapy for acute myocardial infarction, *N Engl J Med* (1994) **331**:1136–42.

66. Echt DS, Liebson PR, Mitchell LB et al and the CAST Investigators, Mortality and morbidity in patients receiving encainide flecainide or placebo: the Cardiac Arrhythmia Suppression trial, *N Engl J Med* (1991) **324**:781–8.

67. Kennedy H, Brooks MM, Barker AH et al, Beta-blocker therapy in the Cardiac Arrhythmia Suppression Trial, *Am J Cardiol* (1994) **74**:674–80.

68. Kjekshus J, Gilpin J, Cali G et al, Diabetic patients and beta-blockers after acute myocardial infarction, *Eur Heart J* (1990) **11**: 43–50.

69. Jonas M, Reicher-Reiss H, Boyko V et al, Usefulness of beta-blocker therapy in patients with non-insulin dependent diabetes mellitus and coronary artery disease, *Am J Cardiol* (1996) **77**:1273–7.

70. Yusuf S, Peto R, Lewis J, Collins R, Sleight P, Beta blockade during and after myocardial infarction. An overview of the randomized trials, *Prog Cardiovasc Dis* (1985) **27**:335–71.

71. Held PH, Yusuf S, Furberg C, Calcium channel blockers in acute myocardial infarction and unstable angina: an overview, *Br Med J* (1989) **299**:1187–92.

72. Psaty BM, Heckbert SR, Koepsell TD et al, The risk of myocardial infarction associated with antihypertensive drug therapies, *JAMA*, (1990) **274**:620–5.

73. Beevers DG, Sleight P, Short acting dihydropyridines (vasodilating) calcium channel blockers for hypertension: is there a risk? *Br Med J* (1996) **312**:1143–5.

74. Opie LH, Messerlie FH. Nifedipine and mortality. Grave defects in the dossier, *Circulation* (1995) **92**:1068–73.

75. Horton R, Spinning the risks and benefits of calcium antagonists, *Lancet* (1995) **346**:586–7.

76. Alderman MH, Cohen H, Roque R, Madhaven S, Effect of long acting and short acting calcium antagonists on cardiovascular outcomes in hypertensive patients, *Lancet* (1997) **349**:594–8.

77. McMurray J, Murdoch D, Calcium antagonist controversy: the long and the short of it? *Lancet* (1997) **349**:585–6.

77a. Staessen JA, Fagard R, Thisj L et al, Randomized double blind comparison of placebo and active treatment for older patients with isolated systolic hypertension, *Lancet* (1997) **350**:757–64.

78. Henry PD, Atherogenesis, calcium and calcium antagonist, *Am J Cardiol* (1990) **66**:31–61.

79. Venkata C, Ram S, Anti-atherosclerotic and vasculoprotective actions of calcium antagonists, *Am J Cardiol* (1990) **66**:29–32.

80. Fleckenstein-Grun G, Frey M, Thimm F et al, Differentiation between calcium and cholesterol-dominated types of arteriosclerotic lesions: antiarteriosclerotic aspects of calcium antagonists, *J Cardiovasc Pharmacol* (1991) **18** (suppl 6):S1–9.

81. Fleckenstein-Grun G, Frey M, Thimm F et al, A calcium overload – an important cellular mechanism in hypertension and arteriosclerosis, *Drugs* (1992) **44** (suppl 1):23–30.

82. Keogh A, Schroeder JS, A review of calcium antagonists and atherosclerosis, *J Cardiovasc Pharmacol* (1990) **16** (suppl 6):S28–35.

83. Schneider W, Kober G, Roebruck P et al, Retardation of development and progression of coronary atherosclerosis: a new indication for calcium antagonists? *Eur J Clin Pharmacol* (1990) **39** (suppl 1):S17–23.

84. Parmley W, Vascular protection from atherosclerosis: potential of calcium antagonists, *Am J Cardiol* (1990) **66**:16–22.

85. Dale J, Landmark KH, Mchure E, The effects of nifedipine a calcium antagonist on platelet function, *Am Heart J* (1983) **105**:103–5.

86. Ferrari R, Visioli I, Protective effects of calcium antagonists against ischaemic and reperfusion damage, *Drugs* (1991) **42** (suppl 1):14–27.

87. Nayler WG, Basic mechanisms involved in the protection of the ischaemic myocardium: the role of calcium antagonists, *Drugs* (1991) **42** (suppl 2):21–7.

88. Skolnick AE, Frishman WH, Calcium channel blockers in myocardial infarction, *Arch Intern Med* (1989) **149**:1669–77.

89. Loaldi A, Polese A, Montorsi P et al, Comparison of nifedipine, propranolol and ISDN on angiographic progression and regression of coronary arterial narrowings in angina pectoris, *Am J Cardiol* (1981) **64**:433–9

90. The INTACT Study Group, Retardation of angiographic progression of coronary disease with nifedipine. Results of INTACT, *Lancet* (1990) **335**:3–7.

91. Waters D, Lesperance J, Francetich M et al, A controlled clinical trial to assess the effect of calcium antagonist upon the progression of coronary atherosclerosis, *Circulation* (1990) **82**:1940–53.

92. Sirnes PA, Overskeid K, Pedersen TR et al, Evaluation of infarct size during the early use of nifedipine in patients with acute myocardial infarction: The Norwegian Nifedipine Multicentre Trial, *Circulation* (1984) **70**:638–44.

93. Muller JE, Morrison J, Stone PH et al, Nifedipine therapy for patients with threatened and acute myocardial infarction: a randomised double-blind, placebo controlled comparison, *Circulation* (1984) **69**:740–7.

94. Wilcox RG, Hampton JR, Banks DC et al, Trial of early nifedipine in acute myocardial infarction: the TRENT Study, *Br Med J* (1986) **293**:1204–7.

95. Branagan JP, Walsh K, Kelly P et al, Effect of early treatment with nifedipine in suspected acute myocardial infarction, *Eur Heart J* (1986) **7**:859–65.

96. Erbel R, Pop T, Meinertz T et al, Combination of calcium channel blocker and thrombolytic therapy in acute myocardial infarction, *Am Heart J* (1988) **115**:529–38.

97. Report of the Holland Interuniversity Nifedipine/Metoprolol Trial (HINT) Research Group, Early treatment of unstable angina in the coronary care unit: a randomised, double blind, placebo controlled comparison of recurrent ischaemia in patients treated with nifedipine or metoprolol or both, *Br Heart J* (1986) **56**:400–13.

98. Walker L, MacKenzie G, Adgey J, Effect of nifedipine in the early phase of acute myocardial infarction on enzymatically estimated infarct size and arrhythmias, *Br Heart J* **57**:83–4.

99. Gottileb SO, Becker LC, Weiss JL et al, Nifedipine in acute myocardial infarction: assessment of left ventricular function, infarct size and infarct expansion. A double blind, randomised, placebo controlled trial *Br Heart J* (1988) **59**:411–18.

100. Israeli SPRINT Study Group, Secondary prevention reinfarction Israeli nifedipine trial (SPRINT). A randomised intervention trial of nifedipine in patients with acute myocardial infarction, *Eur Heart J* (1988) **9**:354–64.

101. SPRINT Study Group, Secondary prevention re-infarction Israeli nifedipine trial (SPRINT II), *Eur Heart J* (1988) **9** (suppl 1):350.

102. Borhani NO, Mercuri M, Borhani PA et al. Final outcome results of the multicentre isradipine diuretic. Atheroscrelosis study (MIDAS), *JAMA* (1996) **276**:785–91.

103. Midtbo KA, Effects of long term verapamil therapy on serum lipids and other metabolic parameters, *Am J Cardiol* (1990) **66**:13-I–15-I.

104. Kober G, Schneider W, Kaltenback M, Can the progression of coronary sclerosis be influenced by calcium antagonists? *J Cardiovasc Pharmacol* (1989) **13** (suppl 4):S2–6.

105. Magnani B, Dal-Palu C, Zanchetti A (Verapamil in Hypertension Atherosclerosis Study Investigators), Preliminary clinical experience with calcium antagonists in atherosclerosis, *Drugs* (1992) **44** (suppl 1):128–33.

106. Crea F, Deanfield J, Crean P et al, Effects of verapamil in preventing early postinfarction angina and reinfarction, *Am J Cardiol* (1985) **55**:900–4.

107. Bussman WD, Seher W, Gruengras M, Reduction of creatinine kinase and creatinine kinase-MB indexes of infarct size by intravenous verapamil, *Am J Cardiol* (1984) **54**:1224–30.

108. Danish Study Group on Verapamil in Myocardial Infarction, The Danish studies on verapamil in myocardial infarction, *Br J Clin Pharmacol* (1986) **21**:197S–204S.

109. Danish Study Group on Verapamil in Myocardial Infarction, The effect of verapamil on mortality and major events after acute myocardial infarction. The Danish Verapamil Infarction Trial II (DAVIT II), *Am J Cardiol* (1990) **66**:779–85.

110. Rengo F, Carbonin P, Pahor M et al, A controlled trial of verapamil in patients after acute myocardial infarction: results of the Calcium Antagonist Reinfarction Italian Study (CRIS) *Am J Cardiol* (1996) **77**:365–9.

111. Gibson RS, Boden WE, Theroux P et al, Diltiazem and reinfarction in patients with non Q wave myocardial infarction: results of a double blind randomized multicentre trial, *N Engl J Med* (1986) **315**:423–9.

112. Zannad F, Amor M, Karcher G et al, Effect of diltiazem on myocardial infarct size estimated by enzyme release, serial thallium-201 single-photon emission computed tomography and radionuclide angiography, *Am J Cardiol* (1988) **61**:1172–7.

113. The Multicentre Diltiazem Post-Infarction Trial Research Group, The effect of diltiazem on mortality and reinfarction after myocardial infarction, *N Engl J Med* (1988) **319**:385–92.

114. Boden WE, Krone RJ, Kleiger RE et al, Diltiazem reduces long-term cardiac event rate after non Q wave infarction: Multicentre Diltiazem Post Infarction Trial (MDPIT), *Circulation* (1988) **78** (suppl 2):**II-96** (Abstract).

115. Pahor M, Guralnik JM, Furberg CD, Carbonin P, Havlik RJ, Risk of gastrointestinal haemorrhage with calcium antagonists in hypertensive patients over 67 years old, *Lancet* (1996) **347**:1061–5.

116. Pahor M, Guralnik JM, Salive ME, Corti MC, Carbonin P, Havlik RJ, Do calcium channel blockers increase the risk of cancer? *Am J Hypertens* (1996) **9**:695–9.

117. Jick H, Jick SS, Derby LE, Validation of information recorded on general practitioner based computerised data resource in the United Kingdom, *Br Med J* (1991) **302**:766–8.

118. Jick H, Jick S, Derby LE, Vasilakis C, Myers MW, Meler CR, Calcium channel blockers and risk of cancer, *Lancet* (1997) **349**:525–8.

119. Garg R, Yusuf S, Overview of randomized trials of angiotensin-converting enzyme inhibitors on mortality and morbidity in patients with heart failure, *JAMA* (1995) **273**:1450–6.

120. Latini R, Maggioni AP, Flather M, Sleight P, Tognoni G, ACE inhibitor use in patients with myocardial infarction: summary of evidence from clinical trials, *Circulation* (1995) **92**:3132–7.

121. Lonn EM, Yusuf S, Jha P et al, Emerging role of angiotensin-converting enzyme inhibitors in cardiac and vascular protection, *Circulation* (1994) **90**:2056–69.

122. Francis GS, Cohn JN, Heart failure: mechanisms of cardiac and vascular dysfunction and the rationale for pharmacologic intervention, *FASEB J* (1990) **4**:3068–75.

123. Francis G, Benedict C, Johnstone DE et al, Comparison of neuroendocrine activation in patients with left ventricular dysfunction with and without congestive heart failure: a substudy of the Studies of Left Ventricular Dysfunction (SOLVD), *Circulation* (1990) **82**:1724–9.

124. Goldsmith SR, Francis G, Cohn JN, Attenuation of the pressor response to intravenous furosemide by angiotensin converting enzyme inhibition in congestive heart failure, *Am J Cardiol* (1989) **64**:1382–5.

125. Ray S, McMurray J, Dargie HJ, ACE inhibition after myocardial infarction. In: Cleland JGF, ed, *The Clinician's Guide to ACE Inhibitors* (Churchill Livingstone: Edinburgh, 1993) 135–49.

126. Tan LB, Jalil JE, Pick R, Janicki JS, Webber KT, Cardiac myocyte necrosis induced by angiotensin II, *Circ Res* (1991) **69**:1185–95.

127. Cohn JN, Johnson G, Ziesche S et al, A comparison of enalapril with hydrazaline-isosorbide dinitrate in the treatment of chronic congestive heart failure, *N Engl J Med* (1991) **325**:303–10.

128. Raynolds MV, Bristow MR, Bush EW et al, Angiotensin-converting enzyme DD genotype in patients with ischaemic or idiopathic dilated cardiomyopathy *Lancet* (1993) **342**:1073–5.

129. Sanderson JE, Young RP, Yu CM, Chan S, Critchley JAJH, Woo KS, Lack of association between insertion/deletion polymorphism of the angiotensin-converting enzyme gene and end-stage heart failure due to ischemic or idiopathic dilated cardiomyopathy in the Chinese, *Am J Cardiol* (1996) **77**:1008.

130. Andersson B, Sylven C, The DD genotype of the angiotensin-converting enzyme gene is associated with increased mortality in idiopathic heart failure, *J Am Coll Cardiol* (1996) **28**:162–7.

131. Hokimoto S, Yasue H, Fujimoto K et al Expression of angiotensin-converting enzyme in remaining viable myocytes of human ventricles after myocardial infarction *Circulation* (1996) **94**:1513–18.

132. Pinto YM, van Gilst WH, Kingma JH, Schunkert H, for the Captopril and Thrombolysis Study Investigators, Deletion-type allele of the angiotensin-converting enzyme gene is associated with progressive ventricular dilation after anterior myocardial infarction, *J Am Coll Cardiol* (1995) **25**:1622–6.

133. Ohmichi N, Iwai N, Nakamura Y, Kinoshita M, The genotype of the angiotensin-converting enzyme gene and global left ventricular dysfunction after myocardial infarction, *Am J Cardiol* (1995) **76**:326–9.

134. Samani NJ, O'Toole L, Martin D et al, Insertion/deletion polymorphism in the angiotensin-converting enzyme gene and risk of and prognosis after myocardial infarction, *J Am Coll Cardiol* (1996) **28**:338–44.

135. Samani NJ, Thompson JR, O'Toole L, Channer K, Woods KL, A meta-analysis of the association of the deletion allele of the angiotensin-converting enzyme gene with myocardial infarction, *Circulation* (1996) **94**:708–12.

136. Tiret L, Bonnardeaux A, Poirier O et al, Synergistic effects of angiotensin-converting enzyme and angiotensin-II type 1 receptor gene polymorphisms on risk of myocardial infarction, *Lancet* (1994) **344**:910–14.

137. Katsuya T, Koike G, Yee TW et al, Association of angiotensinogen gene T235 variant with increased risk of coronary heart disease, *Lancet* (1995) **345**:1600–3.

138. Alderman MH, Madhavan SH, Ooi WL et al, Association of the renin–sodium profile with the risk of myocardial infarction in patients with hypertension, *N Engl J Med* (1991) **324**:1098–104.

139. Meade TW, Cooper JA, Peart WS, Plasma renin activity and ischemic heart disease, *N Engl J Med* (1993) **329**:616–19.

140. Pfeffer MA, Braunwald E, Moye LA et al, Effect of captopril on mortality and morbidity in patients with left ventricular dysfunction after myocardial infarction: results of the Survival and Ventricular Enlargement Trial, *N Engl J Med* (1992) **327**:669–77.

141. Yusuf S, Pepine CJ, Garces C et al, Effect of enalapril on myocardial infarction and unstable angina in patients with low ejection fractions, *Lancet* (1992) **340**:1173–8.

142. Ridker PM, Gaboury CL, Conlin PR, Seely EW, Williams GH, Vaughan DE, Stimulation of plasminogen activator inhibitor *in vivo* by infusion of angiotensin II: evidence of a potential interaction between the renin–angiotensin system and fibrinolytic function, *Circulation* (1993) **87**:1969–73.

143. Wright RA, Flapan AD, Alberti KGM, Ludlam CA, Fox KAA, Effects of captopril therapy on endogenous fibrinolysis in men with recent, uncomplicated myocardial infarction, *J Am Coll Cardiol* (1994) **24**:67–73.

144. Jansson JH, Boman K, Nilsson TK, Enalapril related changes in the fibrinolytic system in survivors of myocardial infarction, *Eur J Clin Pharmacol* (1993) **44**:485–8.

145. Roubin GS, Cannon AD, Agrawal SK et al, Intracoronary stenting for acute and threatened closure complicating percutaneous transluminal coronary angioplasty, *Circulation* (1992) **85**:916–27.

146. McMurray J, Dargie HJ, Hall AS et al, ACE inhibitors for myocardial infarction and unstable angina, *Lancet* (1992) **340**:1547–9.

147. Mancini GBJ, Henry GC, Macaya C et al, Angiotensin-converting enzyme inhibition with quinapril improves endothelial vasomotor dysfunction in patients with coronary artery disease. The TREND (Trial on Reversing Endothelial Dysfunction) Study *Circulation* (1996) **94**:258–65.

148. The CONSENSUS Trial Group, Effect of enalapril on mortality in severe congestive heart failure: results of the Cooperative North Scandinavian Enalapril Survival Study (CONSENSUS), *N Engl J Med* (1987) **316**:1429–35.

149. Cohn JN, Johnson G, Ziesche S et al, Effect of enalapril on survival in patients with reduced left ventricular ejection fractions and congestive heart failure, *N Engl J Med* (1991) **325**:293–302.

150. Cohn JN, Archibald DG, Ziesche S et al, Effect of vasodilator therapy on mortality in chronic congestive heart failure: results of a Veterans Administration Cooperative Study *N Engl J Med* (1986) **314**:1547–52.

151. The SOLVD Investigators, Effect of enalapril on mortality and development of heart failure in asymptomatic patients with reduced left ventricular ejection fractions and congestive heart failure, *N Engl J Med* (1992) **327**:685–91.

152. The Acute Infarction Ramipril Efficacy (AIRE) Study Investigators, Effect of ramipril on mortality and morbidity of survivors of acute myocardial infarction with clinical evidence of heart failure, *Lancet* (1993) **342**:821–8.

153. Term Evaluation (SMILE) Study Investigators, The effect of angiotensin-converting enzyme inhibitor zofenopril on mortality and morbidity after anterior myocardial infarction, *N Engl J Med* (1995) **332**:80–5.

154. Kober L, TorpPedersen C, Carlsen JE et al, A clinical trial of the angiotensin-converting enzyme inhibitor trandolapril in patients with left ventricular dysfunction after myocardial infarction, *N Engl J Med* (1995) **333**:1670–6.

155. Swedberg K, Held P, Kjekshus J, Rasmussen K, Ryden L, Wedel H for the CONSENSUS II Study Group, Effects of early administration of enalapril on mortality in patients with acute myocardial infarction, *N Engl J Med* (1992) **327**:678–84.

156. Devita C, Fazzini PF, Geraci E et al, Gruppo Italiano per lo Studio della Sopravvivenza nell'Infarto Miocardico, GISSI-3: effects of lisinopril and transdermal glyceryl trinitrate singly and together on

6–week mortality and ventricular function after acute myocardial infarction.

157. ISIS-4 (Fourth International Study of Infarct Survival) Collaborative Group. ISIS-4: a randomised factorial trial assessing early oral captopril, oral mononitrate, and intravenous magnesium sulphate in 58,050 patients with suspected acute myocardial infarction, *Lancet* (1995) **345**:669–85.

158. Flaxon DP, on behalf of the Mullticenter American Research trial with Cilazapril after Angioplasty to prevent Transluminal Coronary Obstruction and Restenosis (MARCATOR) Study Group, Effect of high dose angiotensin-converting enzyme inhibition on restenosis: final results of the MARCATOR study, a multicenter, double-blind, placebo-controlled trial of cilazapril, *J Am Coll Cardiol* (1995) **25**:362–9.

159. The Multicenter European Research trial with Cilazapril after Angioplasty to prevent Transluminal Coronary Obstruction and Restenosis (MERCATOR) Study Group, Does the new angiotensin converting enzyme inhibitor cilazapril prevent restenosis after percutaneous transluminal coronary angioplasty? Results of the MERCATOR Study: a multicenter, randomized, double-blind placebo-controlled trial, *Circulation* (1992) **86**:100–10.

160. Lees R, Dinsmore RE, Can ACE inhibitors alter the course of coronary heart disease? Rationale and protocol for QUIET, *J Cardiovasc Pharmacol* (1992) **20** (suppl B):S33–5.

161. Texter M, Lees RS, Pitt B, Dinsmore RE, Uprichard ACG, The Quinapril Ischemic Event Trial (QUIET) design and methods: evaluation of chronic ACE inhibitor therapy after coronary artery intervention, *Cardiovasc Drugs Ther* (1993) **7**:273–82.

162. Consensus Conference, Lowering blood cholesterol to prevent heart disease, *JAMA* (1985) **253**:2080–6.

163. Leren P, Comparison of effects on lipid metabolism of antihypertensive drugs with alpha and beta adrenergic antagonist properties, *Am J Med* (1987) **82** (suppl 1A):31–5.

164. Kincaid-Smith P, Alpha$_1$-blockers, their antihypertensive efficacy and effects on lipids and lipoproteins, *J Hum Hypertens* (1989) **2** (suppl 2):75–83.

165. Grimm R, Thiazide diuretics and selective alpha blockers: comparison of use in antihypertensive therapy including possible differences in coronary heart disease risk reduction, *Am J Med* (1987) **82** (suppl 1A):26–30.

166. Leren P, Foss PO, Helgeland A et al, Effects of propranolol and prazosin on blood lipids, *Lancet* (1980) **ii**:4–6.

167. Lowenstein J, Neusy AJ, Effects of prazosin and propranolol on serum lipids in patients with essential hypertension, *Am J Med* (1984) **76** (suppl 2A):79–84.

168. Rouffy J, Jaillard J, Effects of two antihypertensive agents on lipids, lipoproteins A and B, *Am J Med* (1986) **80** (suppl 2A):100–3.

169. Krone W, Nagele J, Metabolic changes during antihypertensive therapies, *J Hum Hypertens* (1989) **3** (suppl 2):69–74.

170. Frick MH, Haittunen P, Himanen P et al, A long term double blind comparison of doxazosin and atenolol in patients with mild to moderate essential hypertension, *Br J Clin Pharmacol* (1986) **21** (55):S6–12.

171. Castrigano R, D'Engelo A, Pati T et al, A single-blind study of doxazosin in the treatment of mild-to-moderate essential hypertensive patients with concomitant noninsulin-dependent diabetes mellitus, *Am Heart J* (1988) **116**:1778–84.

172. Lehtonen A, Finnish Multicentre Study Group, Lowered levels of serum insulin, glucose and cholesterol in hypertensive patients during treatment with doxazosin, *Curr Ther Res* (1990) **121**:251–60.

173. Feher MD, Henderson AD, Wadsworth J et al, Alpha-blocker therapy; a possible advance in the treatment of diabetic hypertension – results of a cross-over study of doxazosin and atenolol monotherapy in hypertensive non-insulin dependent diabetic subjects, *J Hum Hypertens* (1990) **4**:571–7.

174. Leren P, The cardiovascular effects of alpha-receptor blocking agents, *J Hypertens* (1992) **10** (suppl 3):S11–14.

175. Bell FP, Effects of antihypertensive agents propranolol, metoprolol, nadolol, prazosin and chlorthalidone on LCAT activity in rabbit and rat aortas and in LCAT activity in human plasma in vitro, *J Cardiovasc Pharmacol* (1985) **7**:437–42.

176. Leren NP, Doxazosin low-density lipoprotein receptor activity, *Acta Pharmacol Toxicol* (1985) **56**:269–72.

177. Krone W, Muler-Wieland D, Nagele H et al, Effects of adrenergic antihypertensives and Ca on LDL receptor synthesis in human mononuclear leukocytes, *Arteriosclerosis* (1985) **5**:542a.

178. Ferrannini E, Buzzigoli G, Bonadonna R et al, Insulin resistance in essential hypertension, *N Engl J Med* (1987) **317**:350–7.

179. Pollare T, Lithell H, Selinus I et al, Application of prazosin is associated with an increase in insulin sensitivity in obese patients with hypertension, *Diabetologia* (1988) **31**:415–20.

180. Lehtonen A, the Finnish Multicentre Study Group, Doxazosin effects on the insulin and glucose in hypertensive patients, *Am Heart J* (1991) **121**:1307–11.

181. Leenen FH, Smith DL, Farkas RM et al, Vasodilators and regression of left ventricular hypertrophy. Hydralazine versus prazosin in hypertensive humans, *Am J Med* (1987) **82**:969–78.

182. Agabiti-Rosei E, Muiesan ML, Rissoni D et al, Reduction of left ventricular hypertrophy after long term antihypertensive treatment with doxazosin, *J Hum Hypertens* (1992) **6**:9–15.

183. Yasumoto K, Takata M, Toshida K et al, Reversal of left ventricular hypertrophy by terazosin in hypertensive patients, *J Hum Hypertens* (1990) **4**:13–18.

184. Hernandez RH, Carvajal AR, Pajuelo JG et al, The effect of doxazosin on platelet aggregation in normotensive subjects and patients with hypertension: an in-vitro study, *Am Heart J* (1991) **121**:389–94.

185. Jansson JH, Johansson B, Boman K et al, Effects of doxazosin and atenolol on the fibrinolytic system in patients with hypertension and elevated serum cholesterol, *Eur J Clin Pharmacol* (1991) **40**:321–6.

186. Lytle TB, Coles SJ, Waite MA, A multicentre hospital study of the efficacy and safety of terazosin and its effects on the plasma cholesterol levels of patients with essential hypertension, *J Clin Pharm Ther* (1991) **16**:263–73.

187. Neaton JD, Gumm RH, Prineas RJ et al, Treatment of Mild Hypertension Study: final results *JAMA* (1993) **270**:713–24.

188. Furberg CD, Yusuf S, Effects of drug therapy on survival in chronic congestive heart failure, *Am J Cardiol* (1988) **62**:41A–45A.

189. Murrell W, Nitroglycerine as a remedy for angina pectoris, *Lancet* (1879) **1**: 113–15.

190. Kendall MJ, Long term therapeutic efficacy with once-daily isosorbide-5-mononitrate (Imdur), *J Clin Pharm Ther* (1990) **15**:169–85.

191. Olsson G, Allgen J, Prophylactic nitrate therapy in angina pectoris: possibilities to optimise treatment, *Can J Cardiol* (1993) **9** (suppl A):1A–5A.

192. Yusuf S, Collins R, McMahon S et al, Effects of intravenous nitrates on mortality in acute myocardial infarctions: an overview of the randomised trials, *Lancet* (1988) **ii**:1088–92.

193. Abrams J, Hemodynamic effects of nitroglycerin and long acting nitrates, *Am Heart J* (1985) **110**: 216–24.

194. Jugdutt BI, Role of nitrates after acute myocardial infarction, *Am J Cardiol* (1992) **70**:82B–87B.

195. Abrams J, Mechanisms of action of the organic nitrates in the treatment of myocardial ischaemia, *Am J Cardiol* (1992) **70**:30B–42B.

196. Yeung AC, Vekshtein VI, Krantz DS et al, The effects of atherosclerosis on the vasomotor response of coronary arteries to mental stress *N Engl J Med* (1991) **325**:1551–6.

197. Lam JYT, Chesebro JH, Fuster V, Platelets, vasoconstriction and nitroglycerin during arterial wall injury, *Circulation* (1988) **78**:712–16.

198. Johnstone M, Lam JYT, Waters D, The antithrombotic action of nitroglycerin: cyclic GMP as a potential mediator, *J Am Coll Cardiol* (1989) **13**:231 (Abstract).

199. Diodati J, Theroux P, Latour JG et al, Effects of nitroglycerin at therapeutic doses on platelet aggregation in unstable angina pectoris and acute myocardial infarction, *Am J Cardiol* (1990) **66**:683–8.

200. Tofler GH, Brezinski D, Schufer Al et al, Concurrent morning increase in platelet aggregability and the risk of myocardial infarction and sudden cardiac death, *N Engl J Med* (1987) **316**:1514–19.

201. Mulcahy D, Keegan J, Cunningham D et al, Circadian variation of total ischaemic burden and its alteration with anti-anginal agents, *Lancet* (1988) **ii**:755–8.

202. Jugdutt BI, Warnica JW, Intravenous nitroglycerin therapy to limit myocardial infarct size, expansion and complications: effect of timing, dosage and infarct locations, *Circulation* (1988) **78**:906–19.

203. Humen D, McCormick I, Jugdutt BI, Chronic reduction of left ventricular volumes at rest and exercise in patients treated with nitroglycerin following anterior myocardial infarction, *J Am Coll Cardiol* (1989) **13**:25A.

204. Flaherty JT, Come PC, Baird MG et al, Effects of intravenous nitroglycerin on left ventricular function and ST segment changes in acute myocardial infarction, *Br Heart J* (1976) **38**:612–21.

205. Bussman WD, Passek D, Seidal W et al, Reduction of CK and CK-MB indexes of infarct size by intravenous nitroglycerin, *Circulation* (1981) **63**:615–22.

206. Jaffe AS, Geltman EM, Tiefenbrum AJ et al, Relation of the extent of inferior myocardial infarction with intravenous nitroglycerin: a randomised prospective study, *Br Heart J* (1983) **49**:452–60.

207. Derrida JJR, Sal R, Chiche P, Effects of prolonged nitroglycerin infusion in patients with acute myocardial infarction, *Am J Cardiol* (1978) **41**:407 (abstract).

208. Chiarello M, Gold HK, Leinback RC et al, Comparison between the effects of nitroprusside and nitroglycerin on ischaemic injury during acute myocardial infarction, *Circulation* (1976) **54**:766–73.

209. Mann T, Cohn PH, Holman BI et al, Effects of nitroprusside on regional myocardial blood flow in coronary disease: results in 25 patients and comparison with nitroglycerin, *Circulation* (1978) **57**:732–8.

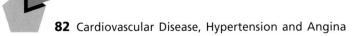

Chapter 3
Metabolic disease
Hyperlipidaemia and diabetes mellitus

Robert Cramb and James Shepherd

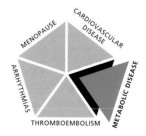

■ HYPERLIPIDAEMIA – INTRODUCTION

Although for many years it was accepted that hypercholestero-laemia was a coronary risk factor and that cholesterol was a major component of atheroma, there was doubt about the clinical benefits of reducing the plasma cholesterol by drugs. Two recently reported studies have shown that reducing the plasma cholesterol in patients known to have coronary artery disease (CAD)[1] and in patients in the general population without gross CAD[2] reduces mortality significantly. A third study has included post-MI patients with a 'normal' plasma cholesterol and, even in these, further lowering of the plasma cholesterol reduced mortality.[3] In each study, the benefits were achieved without causing troublesome or serious adverse effects. It is therefore established that cholesterol-lowering therapy is both safe and effective and must be accepted as a major part of any strategy to reduce coronary mortality.

Although in some ways hyperlipidaemia is like hypertension, a risk factor for CAD which needs to be detected and treated, it differs in at least two main ways. Hyperlipidaemia is a descriptive term for a group of metabolic disorders; it is not a single entity. Also, the drugs currently available to treat hyperlipid-aemia are relatively expensive.

The aim of this chapter is to assist the prescriber to use drugs appropriately to lower the plasma cholesterol of at-risk patients with the aim of reducing the risk of their dying prematurely from CAD.

■ THE RISK FACTOR

The evidence that hyperlipidaemia is a major contributor to the development of CAD is extensive. It may be helpful to classify the evidence into three categories: biological, epidemiological and therapeutic. Some of the key components of each category will be presented briefly.

□ Biological data

Biological data are derived first from animal studies, classically the cholesterol-fed rabbit. These studies show that animals fed a high-cholesterol diet develop lesions in their arteries which closely resemble the atheroma found in humans. Second, pathological studies performed on humans coming to autopsy have shown that cholesterol is a key component of the atheroma and that the extent of the disease correlates with the degree of hypercholesterolaemia recorded during life. Third, patients with familial hypercholesterolaemia who have markedly elevated plasma cholesterol due to a defect in the receptor for low-density lipoprotein (LDL) are more prone to extensive vascular disease which becomes evident at a relatively early age. Fourth, the process of atheroma formation in humans has been extensively investigated. Although the development is not fully understood, it is accepted that LDL will collect in macrophage/monocyte cells (foam cells) and that this process is facilitated if the LDL is oxidized.

☐ Epidemiological data

Countries with a high-fat diet, and whose populations have higher mean plasma cholesterol concentrations have a higher incidence of CAD. The Seven Countries study of Keys[4] was an important study which clearly demonstrated a relationship between hypercholesterolaemia and CAD rates in different countries. This is equally true of communities within countries.

Further, when individuals migrate from countries with a low-fat diet and a low mean plasma cholesterol to countries where the indigenous population consumes more fat, and they adopt the less healthy diet, plasma cholesterol increases, and their coronary risk increases. The effects of migration have been best demonstrated by following a group of Japanese who left their own country to live in Hawaii or the West Coast of the USA.[5] By comparison, countries in which efforts have been made to reduce the fat intake of the population have been rewarded with a decreasing incidence of CAD. Finland is a good example, where a change in the public health policy reducing fat consumed (principally saturated fat) was followed by a reduction in the incidence of CAD.[6]

The largest population groups for which the impact of plasma cholesterol concentrations or CAD risk have been detailed are derived from the USA. The Framingham Study[7] has produced key information based on the long-term follow-up of a community whose coronary risk factors were known and followed. The adverse effects of having a high total plasma cholesterol were established and the prognostic importance of other lipid measurements have been re-evaluated more recently. Analysis of the data from the Multiple Risk Factor Intervention Trial (MRFIT) also showed that those in the highest decile for plasma cholesterol had a four times higher risk of having a coronary event than those in the lowest decile.[8] Furthermore, this study confirmed the marked increase in risk noted when a patient had two or more risk factors, findings which were similar to those in the Framingham Study.

☐ Therapeutic data

The third category is the evidence derived from the results of clinical trials. These will be presented in more detail later in the chapter. However, in the context of making a case for the importance of hyperlipidaemia as a coronary risk factor, the studies which show that lowering cholesterol reduces CAD risk whilst untreated patients continue to be at high risk are perhaps the most persuasive pieces of evidence.

In conclusion, there is no doubt that hypercholesterolaemia is a major cause of CAD and that lowering the plasma cholesterol reduces the risk of suffering from and dying from CAD. However, hyperlipidaemia is a broad term describing a number of metabolic abnormalities involving both cholesterol and triglycerides. A raised plasma cholesterol concentration is associated with increased coronary risk. However, the correlation between total cholesterol and CAD risk is not precise and can only be used as a moderately useful predictor of risk in an individual. A better prediction of risk can be made with the knowledge of the plasma triglyceride concentrations, HDL cholesterol and calculated LDL cholesterol concentrations. It follows therefore that an appreciation of lipid metabolism will allow a more considered assessment of a patient's lipid profile and consequent risk of CAD.

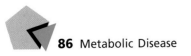

■ THE LIPIDS – THE PROBLEM, THE PATIENT AND THE TREATMENT

□ Lipid metabolism and transport

Lipids are insoluble in water. They are transported in plasma in particles called lipoproteins which contain various proportions of protein, phospholipid, triglyceride and cholesterol. There are a number of different types of lipoproteins, containing varying amounts of these individual constituents. Five major groups of lipoproteins can be recognized (Table 3.1). These are, in increasing density and decreasing size, chylomicrons, very low-density lipoprotein (VLDL), intermediate-density lipoprotein (IDL), low-density lipoprotein (LDL) and high-density lipoprotein (HDL). More detailed analysis of the different lipoprotein fractions makes it possible to determine whether an individual is at greater risk of CAD. At present, the treatment of hyperlipidaemia is based on the measurement of total cholesterol, LDL cholesterol, HDL cholesterol and triglyceride.

Fat from the diet is assembled into large particles which predominantly contain triglycerides and a small amount of cholesterol and apolipoproteins. After expulsion from the thoracic duct into the circulation, they acquire additional apolipoproteins (CII and CIII) from HDL (see below) and they are widely distributed throughout the body in the circulation. Lipoprotein lipase, an enzyme found on capillary endothelium, liberates free fatty acids from triglyceride in chylomicrons, and this process continues, with the chylomicrons reducing in size to form smaller chylomicron remnant particles. Chylomicron remnant particles are taken up by the liver for metabolic destruction.

The liver is responsible for the formation of most of the other lipoprotein particles. This includes the assembly of VLDL particles which again predominantly contain triglyceride, partially synthesized from protein and carbohydrate and also directly transferred from chylomicron remnants. In addition, there are two major apolipoproteins, apolipoprotein B100 and apolipoprotein E, which are responsible for the final metabolic clearance of these particles. Once distributed into the bloodstream, VLDL is metabolized by capillary lipoprotein lipase, releasing free fatty acids from triglyceride with a subsequent reduction in particle size to that of an IDL. This IDL fraction is metabolized by hepatic lipase, which has a similar role to lipoprotein lipase and

Table 3.1 Physicochemical composition of lipid particles.

Name	Density (g/l)	Diameter (nm)	Cholesterol (%)	Triglyceride (%)	Major apolipoprotein(s)
Chylomicrons	<0.95	100–500	3–7	80–95	B_{48} CII CIII
Very low-density lipoproteins (VLDL)	0.95–1.006	25–100	12–18	55–65	B_{100} CII CIII E
Intermediate-density lipoproteins (IDL)	1.006–1.019	10–25	20–25	25–35	B_{100} CII CIII E
Low-density lipoproteins (LDL)	1.019–1.063	2–10	35–40	8–12	B_{100} CIII
High-density lipoproteins (HDL)	1.063–1.210	0.4–1.0	16–24	2–5	AI AII CII CIII

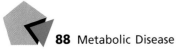

may either be taken up for destruction or released as LDL. LDL may also be produced directly by the liver. This lipoprotein particle, which predominantly contains cholesterol, distributes cholesterol to the peripheral tissues for appropriate metabolism.

LDL is not a single species of particle. It can be relatively large (fluffy and puffy) containing more cholesterol and less protein, or smaller and denser, containing rather less cholesterol and more protein. The major protein component of LDL is apolipoprotein B100. The subclasses of lipoprotein particles have been extensively studied[9,10] and it is clear that those particles which are more dense have a greater propensity to be involved in CAD, and appropriate separation methods have elegantly demonstrated these relationships.

The role of LDL in atheroma formation is well established.[11] However, it is now clear that LDL must be 'altered' to invade the artery wall and form atheroma. Studies by Steinberg et al[12] have shown that chemically modified lipoproteins are a potent stimulus to macrophage activity within endothelial tissues. However, cholesterol is not the only stimulus to atheroma formation within the arterial walls, and it is clear that a number of haemostatic factors, including plasminogen activator inhibitor (PAI-1), fibrinogen and factor VII, all play important roles.[13] Moreover, increased triglyceride concentrations are associated with increased activities of the haemostatic mechanisms, and so raised (and altered) cholesterol concentrations with or without raised triglyceride concentrations are a potent stimulus to atheroma formation. While in the past there was scepticism over the role of triglyceride in CAD, the association with altered haemostasis and observational studies carried out by Assmann and Schulte[14] have altered our views on the risks associated with increased concentrations. There is little doubt that a raised triglyceride concentration must be considered as an important CAD risk factor.

HDLs are a separate group of more protein-dense particles. They are manufactured in the liver and their role is to transport peripheral cholesterol back to the liver. There is an inverse association of HDL-cholesterol concentrations and CAD which has been well established.[7] Although the lipoprotein particles have been described as distinct and mutually exclusive, they do not exhibit metabolic sterility in vivo. They interact, exchanging cholesterol triglyceride and apolipoproteins.

An increased concentration of LDL (and in particular some subfractions), raised plasma triglycerides and a low HDL concentration are all associated with an increased risk of developing CAD. There is good evidence that all three are important risk factors. When a patient is found to have an increased total cholesterol level, it is important to follow this up and review the complete lipid profile, including the triglyceride concentrations and the cholesterol contained within HDL and LDL. For instance, a moderately raised cholesterol level with an increased HDL cholesterol concentration of over 1.5 mmol/l would confer less risk than the same total cholesterol and HDL cholesterol below 1.0 mmol/l. It is mandatory, therefore, to ensure that treatment is planned not only on the basis of risk factors but also on repeated, reliable measurements of plasma total cholesterol, HDL cholesterol, LDL cholesterol and triglycerides.

☐ Determining plasma lipid concentrations

All laboratories undertaking cholesterol testing should be able to reference their cholesterol measurements to a standardized laboratory.[15] Random cholesterol measurements are perfectly acceptable for screening tests and can be performed at any time of the day, with the patient fasting or non-fasting. However, for accurate quantitation of other lipid constituents, patients should have fasted for a minimum of 12 h prior to full lipid quantification. This should include the measurement of cholesterol, triglycerides and HDL cholesterol. A 12-h fast is mandatory in order to ensure that the endogenous production of VLDL is in steady state and to exclude the transient dietary changes in chylomicron formation and metabolism. In some circumstances, notably in alcoholic patients and uncontrolled diabetic patients, chylomicrons may still be found in the plasma and are an indication of the severity of the disease.

Patients should have their blood taken in a standardized way, sitting, resting quietly for at least 5 min, and using the minimum application of a tourniquet to facilitate venous access. Total cholesterol, HDL cholesterol and triglycerides are measured directly, while the LDL cholesterol concentration can be estimated using the Friedewald formula[16] as long as the triglyceride concentrations are no greater than 4.5 mmol/l (Figure 3.1). Direct LDL cholesterol measurements can be made by using ultracentrifugation,[17] though this method is not available in most

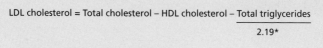

$$\text{LDL cholesterol} = \text{Total cholesterol} - \text{HDL cholesterol} - \frac{\text{Total triglycerides}}{2.19^*}$$

* For measurements in mg/l, divide by 5.0

Figure 3.1 The Friedewald formula.

laboratories. There is a newer method of LDL measurement which relies on antibody complexing apo E-containing lipoproteins, leaving only apo B-containing lipoproteins for measurements of cholesterol. In practice, most patients can easily be assessed and managed with a standard fasting set of lipoprotein measurements which yields three assayed results and one estimated from the formula.

☐ Lipid-lowering drugs

Introduction
The major classes of lipid-lowering agents are shown in Table 3.2. The HMG-CoA drugs are used principally for the treatment of hypercholesterolaemia,[18] though they also have a modest impact on hypertriglyceridaemia. The fibric acid group of drugs can be used for the treatment of isolated hypercholesterolaemia but are particularly effective, and are most commonly used, for the treatment of a patient with a mixed hyperlipidaemia. The nicotinic acid group of drugs is used much less frequently because of their adverse effects as discussed below, and the resins are poorly tolerated by many patients, but they are useful for the correction of isolated hypercholesterolaemia. Combinations of the drugs may be required and are discussed.

Table 3.2 Lipid-lowering drugs.

Drug group	Drug (generic name)	Effect on cholesterol	Effect on triglyceride
HMG-CoA reductase inhibitors	Atorvastatin	↓↓↓	↓↓
	Fluvastatin	↓↓↓	↓
	Pravastatin	↓↓↓	↓
	Simvastatin	↓↓↓	↓
Fibric acid derivatives	Bezafibrate	↓	↓↓↓
	Ciprofibrate	↓	↓↓↓
	Clofibrate*	↓	↓↓↓
	Fenofibrate	↓	↓↓↓
	Gemfibrozil	↓	↓↓↓
Bile acid sequestrants	Cholestyramine	↓	↑↓
	Colestipol	↓	↑↓
Nicotinic acid	Nicotinic acid	↓↓	↓↓
Probucol*	Probucol*	↓	→

*No longer marketed in the United Kingdom.

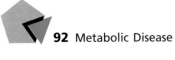

HMG-CoA reductase inhibitors (HMG-CoA)

The HMG-CoA reductase inhibitors (HMG-CoA), also known as the statins, are the most potent cholesterol-lowering drugs. There are a number available with varying degrees of potency. They promote reduction in cholesterol concentrations by decreasing the endogenous synthesis of cholesterol within the liver. This in turn upregulates LDL receptors on the hepatic surface and promotes uptake of cholesterol from the plasma. The reductions in cholesterol concentrations achieved by these drugs are usually between 20 per cent and 40 per cent,[18] but a new statin (atorvastatin)[19] can lower cholesterol by up to 50 per cent. Although their main effect is to decrease plasma cholesterol concentrations, statins reduce triglyceride concentrations. Decreases of up to 15 per cent are reported but atorvastatin can produce reductions of approximately 25 per cent. Increases in HDL cholesterol concentration of up to 5 per cent have been recorded. The side-effect profiles of the statins are similar,[18,19] and include mild gastrointestinal upset, occasional rashes, and, of more concern, a reversible myositis. The myositis may be associated with increases in creatine kinase concentrations in plasma and may occur when a statin is given in combination with a fibric acid derivative[20] or when given to hypothyroid patients.[21] However, the statins have now been used extensively, and in the large clinical trials in which the patients were closely followed, adverse effects were infrequent, occurring in less than 1 per cent of treated patients. Further, they were usually mild and very few patients had to withdraw because of serious unwanted effects.

Fibric acid derivatives

The first clinically important member of the fibric acid family, clofibrate, is now rarely used in the developed countries of the world because of the unfavourable reports it received as a result of the WHO Clofibrate Trial.[22] However, it is still prescribed commonly in Third World countries.

Fibric acid derivatives reduce cholesterol concentrations by 10–25 per cent[18] and triglyceride concentrations by between 20 and 50 per cent. One of their other favourable effects is to increase the concentration of HDL cholesterol by approximately 10 per cent. Of the fibric acid derivatives, gemfibrozil is the only one which has been used in a major primary prevention trial, in which there was only a 10 per cent reduction in cholesterol concentrations but a 34 per cent reduction in total coronary mortality.[23] There were no effects, however, on overall mortality and it was quite clear that most of the beneficial effects were found in the group with a mixed hyperlipidaemia.

The newer drugs, ciprofibrate and fenofibrate, lower the plasma cholesterol concentration more than bezafibrate or gemfibrozil, but to date there are no large studies comparable to the Helsinki Heart Study. Bezafibrate can reduce fibrinogen,[24] while fenofibrate lowers uric acid concentrations by up to 20 per cent.[25]

Side-effects with the fibric acid derivatives are in general more troublesome than those experienced by patients on statins, and include gastrointestinal upset, rashes, which can be particularly unpleasant, headaches and impotence.[18,26]

Anion-exchange resins

There are only two drugs in this group, colestipol and cholestyramine, both of which have been used in primary prevention trials, with cholestyramine being used in a very large cohort primary prevention trial, the Lipid Research Clinics Primary Coronary Prevention Trial.[27,28] Anion-exchange resins work by binding bile salts in the gastrointestinal tract, preventing reabsorption in the enterohepatic circulation, and thus depleting the liver of a cholesterol derivative. The loss of recycled cholesterol stimulates the LDL receptors, and this increases the uptake from plasma and thereby reduces the plasma cholesterol concentration.

Although the anion-exchange resins are successful in lowering plasma cholesterol (by up to 20 per cent), they are marketed as unpalatable powders which have to be dissolved in water or fruit juices. These drugs cause a variety of side-effects, including bloating, indigestion, flatulence, constipation or diarrhoea. These significant gastrointestinal problems usually cause the patient to discontinue the drug. Indeed, in the Lipid Research Clinics trial the aim was to provide patients with an average daily consumption of six sachets (24 g) of cholestyramine. However, most patients could only manage 11 g daily. Further, the anion-exchange resins can also impair the uptake of other drugs.

Nicotinic acid

Nicotinic acid has been used principally in regression trials and shown to be a successful hypolipidaemic agent, reducing plasma cholesterol concentrations by up to 25 per cent and triglyceride concentrations by similar amounts.[18] It also increases HDL concentrations. However, the drug needs to be taken at regular intervals and in large dosage. Its major problems are the development of tolerance and the occurrence of marked, cutaneous flushing. It has been used in a number of studies, particularly the Coronary Drug Project,[29] in which reductions of cholesterol and triglycerides of 10 per cent and 28 per cent, respectively, were noted and this provided benefit in both CAD and overall mortality. This was the first study to show that lipid-lowering therapy could reduce total mortality. Even though it is in widespread use in the USA, few physicians in Europe use this drug.

Probucol
Probucol is a lipid-lowering agent and has antioxidant properties. Its impact on lipids is variable but reductions of as much as 10–20 per cent may be achieved.[18] Data on probucol have shown that it has antioxidant capabilities, but trials in Sweden[30] have shown that, on its own, it does not promote regression. However, when it was used in combination with other lipid-lowering agents, notably the statin group of drugs, there were beneficial effects shown on coronary vasomotion.[31] Despite these favourable data on its use, it is no longer marketed in the UK.

Fish oils
Fish oils contain omega-3 fatty acids (eicosapentanoic and docosahexanoic acids). These agents do not effectively lower cholesterol and may even increase the concentration of LDL cholesterol. However, they have a notable effect on plasma triglyceride concentrations and reduce VLDL particle numbers. Although these drugs are of some use in reducing triglyceride concentrations, they are rarely used.

Combination drug therapy
When the use of a single agent is inadequate, there are a variety of combinations of drug therapy that can be used (Table 3.3). The commonly used combinations include ion-exchange resins with either statins or fibrates. These achieve reductions in total cholesterol concentration much greater than those attained on monotherapy.[18] Combination therapy of statins and fibric acid derivatives is approached rather more warily, because of early

Plasma lipid raised	First-line combination therapy	Second-line combination therapy
Cholesterol	Statin and resin	Fibrate and resin
Triglyceride	Fibrate and resin	Nicotinic acid and resin
Cholesterol and triglyceride	Fibrate and statin	Fibrate and resin

Table 3.3 Drug combination therapy.

descriptions of rhabdomyolysis when these drugs were combined.[32] However, more widespread use of this statin fibrate combination has produced some good results in the treatment of mixed hyperlipidaemia.[33] The use of triple therapy has usually been reserved for patients with very resistant forms of hyper-lipidaemia.[34]

☐ Radical measures for hyperlipidaemia

Two more radical non-drug treatments have been used to treat hyperlipidaemia. They are partial ileal bypass, well described in the POSCH trial,[35] and lipid apheresis. Ileal bypass for reduction of cholesterol is rarely practised now. These bypass operations can cause complications, including impaired absorption of fat-soluble vitamins and loss of trace elements. The POSCH study was the only major long-term controlled trial of this therapy and showed that reduction in cholesterol was associated with a reduced risk of recurrent CAD.

Lipid apheresis is similar to haemodialysis. An extracorporeal circulation is established, with blood entering columns which contain LDL and apo B antibodies. LDL containing apo B is selectively removed from the serum, which is filtered through these columns and returned to the patients. Although this technique lowers LDL concentration effectively and induces regression,[36,37] the costs involved and the specialist nature of the equipment have precluded its introduction into mainstream medical practice. It is, however, of experimental interest and may be particularly valuable in treating patients with resistant forms of heterozygous familial hypercholesterolaemia in addition to those patients with the very rare homozygous familial hyper-cholesterolaemia.

■ CLINICAL DATA

In this section we address the question: *Does lipid-lowering therapy have a clinically relevant and statistically significant effect on vascular disease, particularly in relation to mortality and morbidity?*

The currently available evidence suggests that the beneficial impact of therapy is a direct result of lowering the plasma concentration. The statins, which achieve the greatest reduction in plasma cholesterol, are the drugs for which there is most evidence of efficacy. However, it is possible that further research will suggest that different forms of hyperlipidaemia will require different drug regimens to achieve maximum benefit. It is also possible that some drugs may have a more marked effect on those lipid subfractions which are most atherogenic and may therefore be more cardioprotective. Data of these kind are not yet available, so the protective effects of lipid-lowering drugs as a group will be presented.

□ Primary prevention trials

A number of primary prevention trials have been performed. The early studies included carefully selected patients, have achieved modest reductions in plasma cholesterol (e.g. 5–12 per cent) and have tended to have too few patients followed for too short a time. They have usually shown a reduction in CAD rates (fatal and non-fatal) but have not shown a reduction in overall mortality.

Two of the earlier primary prevention trials merit attention. The Lipid Research Clinic's coronary primary prevention trial[27,28]

was a multicentre, randomized, double-blind study which assessed the impact of cholesterol lowering on CAD events in 3806 asymptomatic men with hypercholesterolaemia unresponsive to diet. The active therapy was cholestyramine and the average length of follow-up was 7.4 years. The compliance was poor, but LDL cholesterol was reduced by 20.3 per cent and there was a 24 per cent reduction in fatal coronary heart disease (CHD) and a 19 per cent reduction in non-fatal myocardial infarction (MI). Fewer patients developed positive exercise tests (25 per cent less) and fewer required coronary artery bypass surgery (21 per cent). However, the overall mortality in the treated and placebo groups was not significantly different.

The Helsinki Heart Study[23] was also a key primary prevention study. In this study, 4081 men with a non-HDL cholesterol concentration above 5.2 mmol/l were randomized to receive gemfibrozil 600 mg twice daily or placebo. On active treatment, LDL was reduced by only 9 per cent but triglycerides were reduced by 40 per cent and HDL was increased by 11 per cent. At 5 years the cumulative rate of cardiac endpoints was 27 per 1000 on gemfibrozil and 44 per 1000 on placebo. There was a 37 per cent reduction in non-fatal MIs and a 25 per cent reduction in CAD deaths. The overall total mortality in the two groups was comparable.

Many accepted that the failure to reduce total mortality was entirely attributable to the lack of power of the study, with the number studied being too small. However, others noted small increases in non-cardiovascular deaths in both of these studies and focused on a non-significant increase in deaths from depression, accidents, suicides and homicide.[38] Though the numbers were small, no consistent pattern emerged and no plausible explanation could be found, it was suggested that some lipid-lowering drugs might have serious adverse effects and/or that lowering plasma cholesterol could in some way be harmful.

The uncertainties and doubts raised by the early primary prevention studies were addressed and answered by the West of Scotland Coronary Prevention Study (WOSCOPS). The key aims of this trial were to determine whether effective reductions in the plasma cholesterol achieved by long-term pravastatin therapy would reduce coronary mortality and total mortality in a group of men with a raised plasma cholesterol. Patients could be entered with stable angina as determined by a Rose questionnaire, but were not selected if they had had a previous MI. The details of the trial design and methodology have been previously presented[2] and are summarized in Figure 3.2.

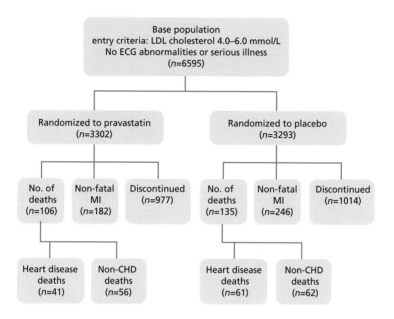

Figure 3.2 WOSCOPS study.

WOSCOPS

The key factors were as follows.

Trial design:	Double-blind, randomized, placebo-controlled parallel-group study.
Patients:	Men (6595) aged 45–64 years Baseline plasma cholesterol >6.5 mmol/l LDL cholesterol >4.5 mmol/l, <6.0 mmol/l Triglycerides <6.0 mmol/l
Treatment:	Pravastatin 40 mg daily or placebo
Numbers:	3302 on pravastatin, 3293 on placebo
Duration:	Average follow-up time 4.9 years

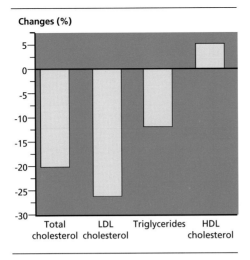

Figure 3.3
WOSCOPS study: impact of pravastatin on plasma lipids (mean percentage changes).

The patients were recruited by specially trained nurses in their local general practitioners' surgeries. Approximately 85 000 men were screened, and after four visits the 6595 who fulfilled the inclusion criteria were randomized. The impact on the patients' plasma lipids are shown in Figure 3.3. This marked reduction in plasma cholesterol, together with a fall in triglycerides and a rise in HDL, achieved a significant reduction in coronary deaths. There was also a decrease in total mortality ($P = 0.051$ by the log rank test, $P=0.039$ using the Cox model) (Figure 3.4). There were no increases in deaths from non-cardiac causes, in contrast to the earlier trials, in fact, there were fewer non-cardiovascular deaths in those on pravastatin. This is a non-significant difference but is important because it shows clearly that neither pravastatin therapy nor cholesterol reduction per se had a significant adverse effect. In subjects who were compliant to therapy (i.e. took more than 75 per cent of the prescribed drug), the benefits were greater. Total mortality in these subjects fell by 32 per cent ($P = 0.015$).

The study was large; and the results were unequivocal and provide data which can be used to assess the efficacy of primary

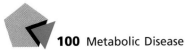

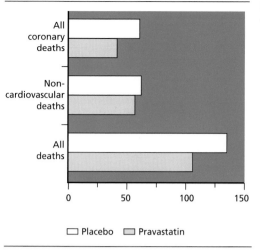

Figure 3.4
WOSCOPS study:
mortality rates.

prevention. Further consideration needs to be given to the clinical implications of these observations, and this is addressed in the next section.

☐ Secondary prevention – angiographic trials

One way of monitoring the efficacy of lipid lowering is to directly measure the diameter of arteries known to have atheroma contained within them and to follow the natural progression of the disease in response to lipid-lowering therapy. There have been a large number of these trials, and the conclusion of them in general is that if cholesterol is lowered the diameter of the coronary arteries will increase (suggesting regression of the atheromatous plaque) or the progressive narrowing of the vessel will be retarded.

Prior to the publication of the clinical trials, these angiographic trials[34,37,39–46] provided valuable scientific evidence that lipid-lowering therapy was effective in altering the course of disease within the artery. The major difficulty with the trials was that although they demonstrated benefit by looking at the difference between progression and regression, the numbers of subjects in the trials were small. Therefore, the relevance of their findings to clinical practice was not clear. Furthermore, the impact on coronary events was much more impressive than the angiographic or ultrasound changes, suggesting that these are poor surrogate markers for measuring the impact of drugs on clinical CAD. Nevertheless, an analysis of these trials[47] revealed an important fact, namely that the percentage reduction in LDL cholesterol correlated better with angiographic outcome than the absolute reduction in LDL cholesterol. No matter what the concentration of cholesterol is, if there is documented CAD active intervention should be considered.

☐ Secondary prevention – clinical trials

An early study, the Coronary Drug Project,[29] recruited 800 men with a history of MI and treated them with a variety of regimens thought to provide benefit, including oestrogen, thyroxine and clofibrate. The use of thyroxine and oestrogen was stopped early on in the trial, as there were excess deaths in the treatment groups. However, niacin (nicotinic acid), which seemed to have little effect initially, was found in the long term to reduce reinfarction rates, but this only became apparent after a 15-year follow-up.

The first secondary prevention study which showed that altering lipid levels could alter the course of disease was the Scandinavian Simvastatin Survival Study usually referred to as the 4S Study.[1] This was a well-planned, well-performed study which, like the WOSCOPS Study, addressed and answered an important question. In 4S, the question was, should patients with known CAD and a moderately raised cholesterol have their cholesterol reduced towards 5.2 mmol/l? The subjects recruited and a summary of outcome is presented in Figure 3.5.

The impact on plasma lipids is shown in Figure 3.6. LDL cholesterol was reduced by 35 per cent. The clinical effects are shown in Figure 3.7. There were 189 (8.5 per cent) and 111 (5.0 per cent) coronary deaths and 256 (11.5 per cent) and 182 (8.2 per cent) total deaths in the placebo and simvastatin groups, respectively. For total mortality, the relative risk on simvastatin was 0.70 (95 per cent CI 0.58–0.85). There were 49 non-cardiovascular deaths

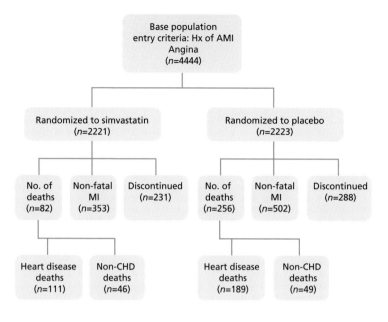

Figure 3.5 4S study.

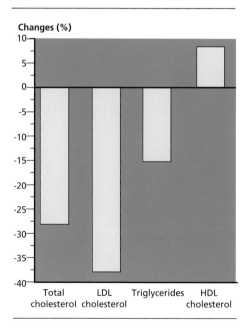

Figure 3.6 4S study: impact of simvastatin on plasma lipids (mean percentage changes).

on placebo and 46 on simvastatin. This trial therefore demonstrated a convincing reduction in coronary deaths and total deaths, with no suggestion of any increase in non-cardiovascular deaths (see Figure 3.7).

The Cholesterol And Recurrent Events (CARE) study has recently been published.[3] This study posed the following question – would lowering cholesterol in patients who had relatively 'normal' cholesterol with CAD influence outcome. A summary of population recruited and the outcome is presented in Figure 3.8.

The impact on plasma lipids is shown in Figure 3.9. LDL cholesterol was reduced by 32 per cent. The clinical effects are shown in Figures 3.8 and 3.10. The primary endpoint in this trial, was death from CAD or non-fatal MI, and there were 274 (13.2 per cent) events on placebo and 212 (10.2 per cent) on active therapy (risk reduction 24 per cent; 95 per cent CI 9–36, $P = 0.03$). There were 196 deaths in the placebo group compared with 180 deaths in the active therapy group (risk reduction 9 per cent; 95 per cent CI to 12–26, $P = 0.37$). An important point of

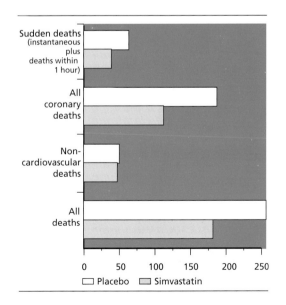

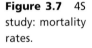

Figure 3.7 4S study: mortality rates.

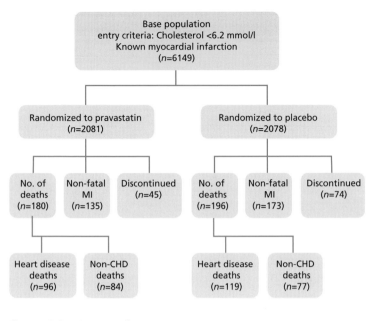

Figure 3.8 CARE study.

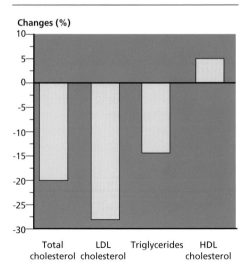

Figure 3.9 CARE study: impact of pravastatin on plasma lipids (mean percentage changes compared to placebo).

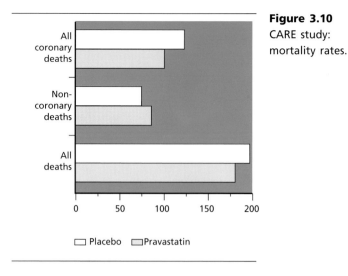

Figure 3.10
CARE study:
mortality rates.

☐ Placebo ☐ Pravastatin

this study is that there appeared to be benefit where the LDL cholesterol was above 3.2 mmol/l. When the LDL cholesterol was below this, intervention did not produce benefit. Further, where the triglyceride concentrations were above 1.6 mmol/l a reduction in events was noted, but this was not significant, suggesting that the type of particle predominating may have an effect on the outcome of treatment.

The trial did show 161 cancers in the placebo group compared with 172 in the pravastatin group. The only cancer that did appear to increase was breast cancer; there were 12 cases in the active therapy group compared with one in the placebo group. All of the cases were non-fatal, with three developing in patients previously known to have the disease, one in a patient with a ductal carcinoma and one in a patient who took active drug for 6 weeks only. This has not occurred in any other major trial and this group of drugs has been extensively investigated. It may well be an isolated random finding, but, like all of these findings, requires long-term surveillance.

Finally, a short mention should be made of the Bezafibrate Coronary Atherosclerosis Intervention Trial (BECAIT). The primary endpoints in this trial[48] were angiographic. All patients

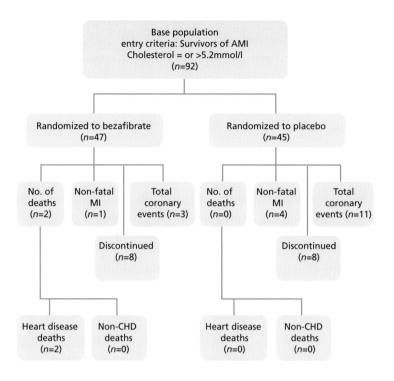

Figure 3.11   BECAIT study.

received diet advice prior to randomization and had angiography upon entry to the study which was repeated at end year 2 and year 5. A summary of this study is shown in Figure 3.11.

In this study the cholesterol and triglyceride concentrations were significantly reduced by 9 per cent and 31 per cent respectively. There was a 0.13-mm difference in the mean lumen diameter of the coronary arteries (95 per cent CI 0.10–0.15; $P = 0.049$), but it is of clinical interest that there was a significant reduction in the cumulative coronary events over the course of the study (3 versus 11 patients; $P = 0.02$) (see Figure 3.11).

The importance of this study is that the triglyceride levels were significantly reduced and this represents a reduction in the

VLDL particle concentrations. Increased VLDL may cause other subtle changes in the particle size of LDL, and this evidence, taken in conjunction with the CARE study, emphasises the need to assess which lipid-lowering agent may provide greatest benefit.

☐ Who should receive lipid-lowering therapy?

There now seems little doubt that raised lipid levels, where the cholesterol level is above 5.2 mmol/l and the patient has documented CAD, should be treated. Benefits will accrue from a reduced incidence of total mortality, and recurrent CAD, especially where the cholesterol concentration is above 6.5 mmol/l. Additionally, patients who have familial hyperlipidaemias, especially familial hypercholesterolaemia, should have therapy.

Where there is still doubt is in the area of primary prevention. The WOSCOPS study has shown that in a high-risk population the incidence of MI is reduced. The overall mortality was also reduced ($P = 0.051$ or $P = 0.039$ depending on the statistical method used) and the reduction was most evident in those who complied with therapy ($P < 0.015$). Further analysis of the WOSCOPS data, taken in conjunction with the results of other trials and the authoritative European Guidelines on CAD,[49,50] suggest that in high-risk individuals the treatment of hyperlipidaemia is of greater benefit than treating mild hypertension in patients of the same age and sex. There is acceptance that to achieve comparable benefit in primary prevention requires three times as many people to be treated as in secondary prevention such as in the 4S study. Naturally, there is debate about this approach and in particular the cut-off point where 'risk' occurs. Ramsey and his colleagues[51] suggest that this should be at 3 per cent/year risk of CAD, whereas the WOSCOPS group feels that this might be more appropriate at 2 per cent/year.[49] Although there are these disagreements, the overriding concern from each of them is that high-risk individuals should be treated. The 'Sheffield' table provides useful succinct guidelines based on readily available information on risk factors on which to base the decision to treat. It is, however, not tested as a tool and takes particular note of economic factors in relation to intervention.[52,53] We should, however, remember that the incidence of CAD is affected by other subtle effects, including ethnic group and social class,[54,55] and any decision to treat should be made on the basis of the needs of the patient, with the recommendations from the various groups being taken into consideration. In practice, a patient with a plasma cholesterol over 6.5 mmol/l who has two other risk factors, one of which could be male gender, should have lipid-lowering therapy. The risk factors documented in the WOSCOPS Study[2,49] included family history, minor ECG changes, hypertension, low HDL and smoking.

☐ What therapy should be given?

Central to any treatment of hyperlipidaemia is attention to the diet of the patient. Some have cast doubt on the efficacy of diet,[56] but others have shown that attention to diet, and, in particular, a reduction of total fat consumed, can lead to modest but clinically significant reductions in cholesterol.[57,58] Where drugs are prescribed and diet ignored, with the consequences of weight gain, the effect of the drug is negated.[59] Diet advice and encouragement to achieve an ideal body mass must be the cornerstone of any therapy that is used to reduce plasma lipids.

The difficulty is the selection of the drugs. Statins are potent and their efficacy has been demonstrated in large clinical trials. There is a lingering doubt that they may not be as good at reducing CAD in patients where the plasma triglyceride concentration is raised.[3] The fibric acid derivatives have been shown to be useful in primary prevention, but do not reduce overall mortality. In secondary prevention there are encouraging data, on fibrates but only in small-scale trials. We need the results of much larger trials that are currently being undertaken to be sure that they are equipotent and as safe as the statins.

Therefore, for pragmatic purposes, statins should be prescribed as first-line therapy to patients who clinically merit their need as long as two criteria are met. These are:

- the total cholesterol is greater than 5.2 mmol/l and/or the calculated LDL cholesterol is greater than 3.2 mmol/l
- the triglyceride concentration is less than 4.0 mmol/l (3 SD above the mean of the WOSCOPS triglyceride levels)

Where the triglyceride concentrations are higher, a fibric acid derivative should be used.

If the statins in maximum dosage do not provide a sufficient reduction in cholesterol, bile acid sequestrants may be added. Fibric acid derivatives can also be used in combination with statins, but much greater care should be taken to detect early side-effect problems. When there are more data on fibric acid derivatives in secondary prevention,[60] these may be drugs of first choice, depending on the overall lipid profile.

■ DIABETES MELLITUS

Insulin-dependent diabetic patients (IDDMs) and non-insulin-dependent diabetic patients (NIDDMs) are more likely to suffer from and die prematurely from a variety of disorders compared with non-diabetics, particularly CAD, cerebrovascular disease and peripheral arterial disease.[61]

For CAD, diabetes is a strong independent risk factor and it is both more common and more severe in diabetic patients. In one large study,[62] 41 per cent of diabetic patients died within 1 year of infarction, with a further 23 per cent experiencing reinfarction, compared with 26 per cent and 14 per cent respectively for non-diabetics. Overall, diabetic males are 2–3 times more likely to die from CAD, whilst diabetic females are at 3–7 times greater risk than their non-diabetic counterparts.[63–66] Following MI, both early and late mortality are higher in diabetic than in non-diabetic patients.[66–69] The increased morbidity and mortality in diabetics have not improved substantially despite recent developments in coronary care, and this suggests that diabetic patients have special problems that, so far, have not been adequately addressed.

Hypertension is twice as common in diabetic individuals[70] and is particularly harmful, since it leads to a worsening of the micro- and macrovascular complications of diabetes[71]. Hypertensive diabetics are more likely to suffer a stroke, and the prognosis is poor[72,73]. The combination of diabetes and hypertension also substantially increases the risk of developing CAD. For any given blood pressure, the presence of diabetes increases the risk of and mortality from cardiovascular disease[74]. Mortality increases with rising blood pressure, but the mortality rate of the non-diabetics

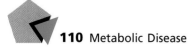

with relatively high blood pressures remains below that of diabetic individuals with low blood pressures,[74].

Hyperinsulinaemia and insulin resistance are associated with hypertension and may have a causative role.[75] Furthermore, high fasting plasma insulin concentrations appear to be an independent risk factor for ischaemic heart disease in men.[76] This could contribute to the increase in risk in both NIDDMs, many of whom have high insulin concentrations, and in the IDDMs, in whom the injection of insulin can produce higher peripheral insulin concentrations than in healthy subjects whose pancreatic insulin production is largely cleared by the liver. However, the potential role of high plasma insulin concentrations is complex and ill understood.

Diabetics, whether they are insulin-dependent or non-insulin dependent, are at increased risk of premature atherosclerosis. The association of premature atherosclerosis with increased serum lipids is well recorded. There is an increased risk of CAD and death for any given level of serum cholesterol in diabetics by comparison to the non-diabetic population.[77] In addition, the serum triglyceride level in diabetic subjects is a good predictor of CAD,[78,79] an association more recently proven in the non-diabetic population.[14]

It is well known that insulin resistance has major effects on lipid metabolism. One of the most significant effects is that there is a predominance of small, dense LDL particles where there is insulin resistance and these particles confer a greater risk of cardiovascular disease.[9,10,80]

A reduction in fibrinolysis is a feature of diabetes,[81,82] and hyperinsulinaemia has been linked with this problem.[83] This has been shown to be due to an increase in circulating PAI-1. There is a strong correlation of PAI-1 concentrations and hyperinsulinaemia, but increased levels of PAI-1 are found in patients who are obese, have raised triglyceride concentrations or have raised blood pressure;[13,84] these are all features of the insulin resistance syndrome.

As a result of all of these effects, the arterial endothelium of a diabetic patient is more susceptible to premature atherosclerosis. In addition, diabetic patients are more susceptible to the effects of increased oxidative stress, non-enzymic glycosylation of protein and increased platelet aggregability.[85–87]. These features of cardiovascular dysfunction reveal why diabetic patients are at greater risk of premature death.

The autonomic neuropathy commonly found in diabetics is a major concern, as it may lead to a reduction in infarction-related pain. Thus silent infarctions are more common in diabetics.[85,88] Furthermore, increased heart rate and decreased vagal tone in diabetics may lead to more extensive infarction and heightened risk of sudden death. Resting heart rates are increased by at least 10 beats per minute and diurnal variability is lost, leaving diabetics at increased risk throughout the 24 h, and in addition it is postulated that increased diastolic flow rates and shear stress exacerbate the endothelial damage.[89-91] Diabetics are also more prone to develop congestive heart failure following MI, possibly due to a specific diabetic cardiomyopathy.[92,93]

The frequency, severity and poor prognosis of coronary events in diabetic patients require that in these patients every effort is made to prevent the first infarction (primary prevention), to reduce the mortality at the time of infarction and to improve the prognosis of the post-MI diabetic patients (secondary prevention).

☐ Primary prevention

Clinical logic would suggest at least three approaches to delay the first infarction in the diabetic patient. First, the lifestyle changes, particularly smoking cessation and weight reduction, which are known to reduce coronary risk in non-diabetic patients should be strongly advised. Second, since disturbed carbohydrate homeostasis is the hallmark of diabetes, strict diabetic control would seem prudent. Third, those drugs discussed elsewhere in this book which have been shown to have a cardioprotective role in diabetics (aspirin, beta-blockers, lipid-lowering therapy, hormone replacement therapy) should be advocated, particularly if there is evidence of their efficacy in diabetic patients.

Scientific support for the above suggestions is surprisingly limited. Further, the lack of data on 'hard' clinical endpoints often leads to decisions being made on the basis of effects on surrogate makers. Drugs are therefore commended or condemned on the basis of biochemical effects or changes in diabetic control rather than on their impact on mortality and morbidity. It would seem more honest to state that lifestyle changes, good diabetic control and the appropriate use of cardioprotective drugs should be considered prudent but unproven.

Managing the acute infarct

Diabetic patients, in spite of the benefits of thrombolysis and optimal care, continue to have a mortality rate twice that of non-diabetic patients matched for age and sex.[67,69,94,95] There are many reasons for this, including autonomic dysfunction,[89,90,91] insulin resistance, low plasma insulin concentrations and high plasma concentrations of non-esterified fatty acids.[95,96] The logic of providing glucose and insulin to correct some of the major metabolic abnormalities has been appreciated for many years. Clinical trial data to support this belief have been lacking until recently, but a trial on 6000 Swedish diabetic patients[97] has now shown convincingly that a glucose–insulin infusion designed to keep the plasma glucose concentration in the range 7–10.9 mmol/l over the first 24 h reduced one year mortality by 29 per cent (95 per cent CI—14–51 per cent) 57 deaths in the intervention group and 82 deaths in the controls ($P = 0.03$).

Secondary prevention

Diabetic patients who survive a myocardial infarct will probably benefit from aspirin therapy and an ACE inhibitor if they have left ventricular dysfunction. For beta-blockers there is some evidence that in clinical trials they improve the prognosis and reduce the mortality rates. Diabetic patients in randomized post-MI trials have been monitored, and those on a beta-blocker have a much greater reduction in mortality than is achieved in non-diabetic patients.[85,98,99] The data from the Norwegian Timolol Study,[100,101] the American BHAT (propranolol) trial[102] and a further study on propranolol reported by Kjekshus et al[98] are presented in Figures 2.7 and 3.12. In addition a recent observational study (noted in the beta-blocker section) revealed that beta-blocker therapy in patients with known CAD is associated with a 44 per cent lower mortality rate.[103] Recent data show that diabetic patients benefit from lipid lowering therapy using a statin. In a sub-group analysis of the 4S study[104] and the CARE Study,[3] diabetics had statistically significant reductions in major coronary events when treated with a statin. Overall mortality in these small sub-groups was (not significantly) reduced but the absolute clinical benefit is cholesterol reduction in diabetics may be better than in non-diabetics since they have a higher absolute risk of recurrent atherosclerotic events.

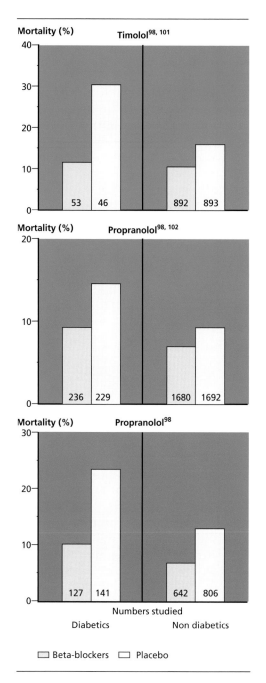

Figure 3.12 The impact of beta-blockers in diabetic and non-diabetic patients – three post-infarct studies.[98,101,102]

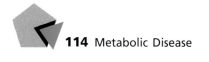

☐ Conclusion

Diabetic patients are a high risk group. Data on how best to reduce the coronary mortality are, however, very sparse. It would seem sensible to advocate the measures found to be effective in non-diabetic patients. In addition since there are clinical trial data indicating efficacy of glucose-insulin infusion, these should form part of the management of the AMI patient and lipophilic beta-blockers and statins part of the management of the post-MI patient.

References

1. The Scandinavian Simvastatin Survival Study Group, Randomised trial of cholesterol lowering in 4444 patients with coronary heart disease: the Scandinavian Simvastatin Survival Study (4S), *Lancet* (1994) **344**:1383–9.

2. Shepherd J, Cobbe SM, Ford I et al, Prevention of coronary heart disease with pravastatin in men with hypercholesterol-aemia, *N Engl J Med* (1995) **333**:1301–7.

3. Sacks FM, Pfeffer MA, Moye LA et al, The effect of pravastatin on coronary events after myocardial infarction in patients with average cholesterol levels, *N Engl J Med* (1996) **335**:1001–9.

4. Keys A, Coronary heart disease – the global picture, *Atherosclerosis* (1975) **22**:149–92.

5. Robertson TL, Kato H, Gordon T et al, Epidemiologic studies of coronary heart disease and stroke in Japanese men living in Japan, Hawaii, and California. Incidence of myocardial infarction and death from coronary heart disease, *Am J Cardiol* (1977) **39**:239–43.

6. Pyörälä K, Salonen JT, Valkonen T, Trends in coronary heart disease mortality and morbidity and related factors in Finland, *Cardiology* (1985) **72**:35–51.

7. Castelli WP, Garrison RJ, Wilson PWF, Abbott RD, Kalousdian S, Kannel WB, Incidence of coronary heart disease and lipoprotein cholesterol levels. The Framingham Study, *JAMA* (1986) **256**:2835–8.

8. Stamler J, Wentworth D, Neaton JD, Is the relationship between serum cholesterol and the risk of premature death from coronary artery disease continuous and graded? *JAMA* (1986) **256**: 2823–8.

9. Austin MA, Breslow JL, Hennekens CH, Buring JE, Willett WC, Krauss RM, Low density lipoprotein subclass patterns and risk of myocardial infarction, *JAMA* (1988) **26**:1917–26.

10. Griffin BA, Freeman DJ, Tait GW et al, Role of plasma triglyceride in regulation of plasma low density lipoprotein (LDL) subfractions: relative contribution of small dense LDL to coronary heart disease risk, *Atherosclerosis* (1994) **106**:241–53.

11. Ross R, The pathogenesis of atherosclerosis. An update, *N Engl J Med* (1986) **314**:488–500.

12. Steinberg D, Parasthasarathy S, Carew TE, Khoo JC, Witzum JL, Beyond cholesterol: modifications of low density lipoprotein that increase its atherogenicity, *N Engl J Med* (1989) **320**:915–23.

13. Fuster V, Fallon JT, Nemerson Y, Coronary thrombosis, *Lancet* (1996) **348** (suppl I):s7–9.

14. Assmann G, Schulte H, The importance of triglycerides: results from the Prospective Cardiovascular Munster (PROCAM) Study, *Eur J Epidemiol* (1992) **8** (suppl):99–103.

15. Packard CJ, Bell MA, Eaton RH, Dagen MM, Cassidy M, Shepherd J, A pilot scheme for improving the accuracy of serum cholesterol measurement in Scotland and Northern Ireland, *Ann Clin Biochem* (1993) **30**:387–93.

16. Friedewald WT, Levy RI, Fredrickson DS, Estimation of the concentration of low-density lipoprotein in plasma without the use of the preparative ultracentrifuge, *Clin Chem* (1972) **18**:499–502.

17. Carlson K, Lipoprotein fractionation, *J Clin Pathol* (1973) **26** (suppl 5):32–7.

18. O'Connor P, Feely J, Shepherd J, Lipid lowering drugs, *Br Med J* (1990) **300**:667–72.

19. Nawrocki JW, Weiss SR, Davidson MH et al, Reduction of LDL cholesterol by 25 per cent to 60 per cent in patients with primary hypercholesterolaemia by Atorvastatin, a new HMG-CoA reductase inhibitor, *Arterioscler Thromb Vasc Biol* (1995) **15**:678–82.

20. Grundy S, HMG-CoA reductase inhibitors for treatment of hypercholesterolaemia, *N Engl J Med* (1988) **319**:24–33.

21. Al-Jubouri MA, Briston PG, Sinclair D, Chinn RH, Young RM, Myxoedema revealed by simvastatin induced myopathy, *Br Med J* (1994) **308**:588.

22. Committee of Principal Investigators, WHO co-operative trial in the primary prevention of ischaemic heart disease using clofibrate, *Br Heart J* (1978) **40**:1069–118.

23. Frick MH, Elo O, Happa K et al, Helsinki Heart Study: primary-prevention trial with gemfibrozil in middle-aged men with dyslipidemia, *N Engl J Med* (1987) **317**:1237–45.

24. Niort G, Bulgarelli A, Cassander M, Pagano G, Effect of short term treatment with bezafibrate on plasma fibrinogen, fibrinopeptide A, platelet activation and blood filterability in atherosclerotic hyper-fibrogenemic patients, *Atherosclerosis* (1988) **71**:113–19.

25. Bastow MD, Durrington PN, Ishola M, Hypertriglyceridaemia and hyperuricaemia: effects of two fibric acid derivatives (bezafibrate and fenofibrate) in a double-blind placebo-controlled trial, *Metabolism* (1988) **37**:217–20.

26. Bharani A, Sexual dysfunction after gemfibrozil, *Br Med J* (1992) **305**:693.

27. The Lipid Research Clinics Program, The Lipid Research Clinics Coronary Primary Prevention Trial results. I Reduction in incidence of coronary heart disease, *JAMA* (1984) **251**:351–64.

28. The Lipid Research Clinics Program, The Lipid Research Clinics Coronary Primary Prevention Trial results. II The relationship of reduction in incidence of coronary heart disease to cholesterol lowering, *JAMA* (1984) **251**:365–74.

29. Coronary Drug Project Group, Clofibrate and niacin in coronary heart disease, *JAMA* (1975) **231**:360–81.

30. Walldius G, Erikson U, Olsson AG et al, The effect of probucol on femoral atherosclerosis: the Probucol Quantitative Regression Swedish Trial (PQRST), *Am J Cardiol* (1994) **74**:875–83.

31. Anderson TJ, Meredith IT, Yeung AC, Frei B, Selwyn AP, Ganz P, The effect of cholesterol-lowering and antioxidant therapy on endothelium-dependent coronary vasomotion, *N Engl J Med* (1995) **332**: 488–93.

32. Pierce LR, Wysoski DK, Gross TP, Myopathy and rhabdomyolysis associated with lovostatin-gemfibrozil combination therapy, *JAMA* (1990) **264**:71–5.

33. Shepherd J, Fibrates and statins in the treatment of hyperlipidaemia: an appraisal of their efficacy and safety, *Eur Heart J* (1995) **16**:5–13.

34. Kane J, Malloy M, Ports T, Phillips N, Diehl J, Havel R, Regression of coronary atherosclerosis during treatment of familial hypercholesterolemia with combined drug regimens, *JAMA* (1990) **264**:3007–12.

35. Buchwald H, Varco R, Matts J et al, Effect of partial ileal bypass surgery on mortality and morbidity from coronary heart disease in patients with hypercholesterolemia. Report of the Program on the Surgical Control of the Hyperlipidemias (POSCH), *N Engl J Med* (1990) **323**:946–55.

36. Schuff-Werner P, Gohlke H, Bartmann U et al, The HELP LDL-apheresis multicentre study; an angiographically assessed trial on the role of LDL-apheresis in the secondary prevention of coronary heart disease. II. Final evaluation of the effect of regular treatment on LDL-cholesterol plasma concentrations and the course of coronary heart disease, *Eur J Clin Invest* (1994) **24**:724–32.

37. Thompson GR, Maher VMG, Matthews S et al, Familial Hypercholesterolaemia Regression Study: a randomized trial of LDL apheresis, *Lancet* (1995) **345**:811–16.

38. Davey-Smith G, Pekkanen J, Should there be a moratorium on lipid-lowering drugs? *Br Med J* (1992) **304**:431–4.

39. Brown G, Albers J, Fisher L et al, Regression of coronary artery disease as a result of intensive lipid lowering therapy in men with high levels of apolipoprotein B, *N Engl J Med* (1990) **323**:1289–98.

40. Watts GF, Lewis B, Brunt JNH et al, Effects on coronary artery disease of lipid-lowering diet, or diet plus cholestyramine, in the St Thomas' Atherosclerosis Regression Study (STARS), *Lancet* (1992) **339**:563–9.

41. Blankenhorn DH, Azen SP, Kramsch DM et al, Coronary angiographic changes with lovostatin therapy. The Monitored Atherosclerosis Regression Study (MARS), *Ann Intern Med* (1993) **119**:969–76.

42. Waters D, Higginson L, Gladstone P et al, Effects of monotherapy with and HMG-CoA reductase inhibitor on the progression of coronary atherosclerosis as assessed by serial quantitative arteriography. The Canadian Coronary Atherosclerosis Intervention Trial, *Circulation* (1994) **89**:959–68.

43. Ornish D, Brown SE, Scherwitz LW et al, Can lifestyle changes reverse coronary artery disease? *Lancet* (1990) **336**:129–33.

44. Haskell W, Alderman E, Fair J et al, Effects of intensive multiple risk factor reduction on coronary atherosclerosis and clinical cardiac events in men and women with coronary artery disease. The Stanford Coronary Risk Intervention Project (SCRIP), *Circulation* (1994) **89**:975–90.

45. MAAS Investigators, Effect of simvastatin on coronary atheroma: the Multicentre Anti-Atheroma Study (MAAS), *Lancet* (1994) **344**:633–8.

46. Pitt B, Mancini J, Ellis SG, Rosman HS, McGovern ME, for the PLAC-1 Investigators, Pravastatin Limitation of Atherosclerosis in the Coronary Arteries (PLAC-1), *JACC* (1994) **26**:131A.

47. Thompson GR, Hollyer J, Waters DD, Percentage change rather than plasma level of LDL-cholesterol determines therapeutic response in coronary heart disease, *Curr Opin Lipidol* (1995) **6**:386–8.

48. Ericsson C, Hamsten A, Nilsson J, Grip L, Svane B, de Faire U, Angiographic assessment of effects of bezafibrate on progression of coronary disease in young male postinfarction patients, *Lancet* (1996) **347**:849–53.

49. West of Scotland Coronary Prevention Group, West of Scotland Coronary Prevention Study: identification of high-risk groups and comparison with other cardiovascular intervention trials, *Lancet* (1996) **348**:1339–42.

50. Pyörälä K, De Backer G, Graham I, Poole-Wilson P, Wood DA, on behalf of the Task Force, Prevention of coronary heart disease in clinical practice: recommendations of the Task Force of the European Society of Cardiology, European Atherosclerosis Society and European Society of Hypertension, *Eur Heart J* (1994) **15**:1300–31.

51. Haq IU, Jackson PR, Yeo WW, Ramsay LE, Cholesterol and prevention of coronary heart disease, *Lancet* (1997) **349**: 210–11.

52. Haq IU, Jackson PR, Yeo WW, Ramsay LE, Sheffield risk and treatment table for cholesterol lowering for primary prevention of coronary heart disease, *Lancet* (1995) **346**:1467–71.

53. Ramsay LE, Haq IU, Jackson PR, Yeo WW, Pickin DM, Payne JN, Targeting lipid-lowering drug therapy for primary prevention of coronary disease: an updated Sheffield table, *Lancet* (1996) **348**: 387–8.

54. Millar WJ, Wigle DT, Socio-economic disparities in risk factors for cardiovascular disease, *Can Med Assoc J* (1986) **134**:127–32.

55. McInnes G, Heart disease in ethnic groups, *Br J Cardiol* (1996) **3**:179–80

56. Ramsay LE, Yeo WW, Jackson PR, Dietary reduction of serum cholesterol concentration: time to think again, *Br Med J* (1991) **303**:953–7.

57. AHA Special Report, Recommendations for the treatment of hyperlipidaemia in adults, *Atherosclerosis* (1984) **4**:445A–68A.

58. Denke MA, Breslow JL, Effects of a low fat diet with and without intermittent saturated fat and cholesterol ingestion on plasma lipid, lipoprotein, and apolipoprotein levels in normal volunteers, *J Lipid Res* (1988) **29**:963–9.

59. Durrington PN, Secondary hyperlipid-aemia. In: Durrington PN, ed. *Hyperlipidaemia: Diagnosis and Management*, 2nd edn (Butterworth-Heinemann Ltd: Cambridge, 1995):291–360.

60. Goldbourt U, Behar S, Reicher-Reiss H et al. Rationale and design of a secondary prevention trial of increasing serum high-density lipoprotein cholesterol and reducing triglycerides in patients with clinically manifest atherosclerotic heart disease (the Bezafibrate Infarction Prevention Trial), *Am J Cardiol* (1993) **71**:909–15.

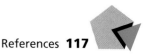

61. Kannel WB, McGee DL. Diabetes and cardiovascular disease. The Framingham Study, *JAMA* (1979) **241** (19):2035–8.

62. Karlson BW, Herlitz J, Halmarson A. Prognosis of acute myocardial infarction in diabetic and non-diabetic patients, *Diabetic Med* (1993) **10**:449–54.

63. Butler W, Ostrander L, Carman W, Lamphiear D, Mortality from coronary heart disease in the Tecumseh study: long term effect of diabetes mellitus, glucose tolerance and other risk factors, *Am J Epidemiol* (1985) **121**:541–7.

64. Kannel W, McGee D, Diabetes and glucose tolerance as risk factors for cardiovascular disease: the Framingham study, *Diabetes Care* (1979) **2**:120–6.

65. Barret-Connor E, Wingard D, Sex differential in ischaemic heart disease mortality in diabetics: a prospective population-based study, *Am J Epidemiol* (1983) **118**:489–96.

66. Manson J, Colditz G, Stampfer M, A prospective study of maturity-onset diabetes and risk of coronary heart disease and stroke in women, *Arch Intern Med* (1991) **151**:1141–7.

67. Rytter L, Froelsen S, Beck-Nielsen H, Prevalence and mortality of acute myocardial infarction in patients with diabetes, *Diabetes Care* (1985) **8**:230–4.

68. Ulvenstam G, Aberg A, Bergstrand R et al, Long-term prognosis after myocardial infarction in men with diabetes, *Diabetes* (1985) **34**:787–92.

69. Zyabetti G, Latinin R, Maggioni AP, Santoro L, Franzosi MG, on behalf of the GISSI-2 investigators. Influence of diabetes on mortality in acute myocardial infarction: data from the GISSI-2 study *J Am Coll Cardiol* (1993) **22**:1788–94.

70. Working Group on Hypertension in Diabetes, Statement on hypertension in diabetes: final report, *Arch Intern Med* (1987) **147**:830–42.

71. Bierman EL, Atherogenesis in diabetes, *Atherosclerosis Thrombosis* (1992) **12**:647–56.

72. Palumbo PJ, Elveback LR, Whisnant JP, Neurologic complications of diabetes mellitus: transient ischaemic attack, stroke and peripheral neuropathy, *Adv Neurol* (1978) **19**:593–601.

73. Asplund K, Hagg E, Helmers C, Lither F, Strand T, Westor PO, The natural history of stroke in diabetic patients, *Acta Med Scand* (1980) **207**:417–24.

74. Poulter N, Hypertension in diabetes and hyperlipidaemia In: Poulter N, Sever P, Thom S, eds. *Cardiovascular Disease. Risk Factors and Intervention*, vol. 13 (Radcliffe Medical Press Ltd, 1993) 305–14.

75. Reaven GM, Lithel H, Landsberg L, Hypertension and associated metabolic abnormalities – the role of insulin resistance and the sympathoadrenal system, *N Engl J Med* (1996) **334**:374–81.

76. Despres J-P, Lamarche B, Mauriege P et al, Hyperinsulinaemia as an independent risk factor for ischemic heart disease, *N Engl J Med* (1996) **334**:952–7.

77. Stamler J, Vaccaro O, Neaton JD, Wentworth D, Diabetes, other risk factors, and 12–year cardiovascular mortality for men screened in the Multiple Risk Factor Intervention Trial, *Diabetes Care* (1993) **16**:434–44.

78. West KM, Ahuja NM, Bennett PH et al, The role of circulating glucose and triglyceride concentrations and their interactions with other 'risk factors' as determinants of arterial disease in nine diabetic population samples from the WHO Multinational Study, *Diabetes Care* (1983) **6**:361–9.

79. Janka HU, Five-year incidence of major macrovascular complications of diabetes mellitus. In: (Janka HU, Mehner H, Standl E, eds.), *Macrovascular Disease in Diabetes Mellitus: Pathogenesis and Prevention*, (Georg Thieme: Stuggart, 1985) 15–19.

80. Austin MA, Selby JV, LDL subclass phenotypes and the risk factors of the insulin resistance syndrome, *Int J Obesity* (1995) **19** (suppl 1):S22–6.

81. Scheider DJ, Nordt TK, Sobel BE, Attenuated fibrinolysis and accelerated atherogenesis in type II diabetic patients, *Diabetes* (1993) **41**(1):1–7.

82. Ostermann H, van de Loo J, Factors of the hemostatic system in diabetic patients. A survey of controlled studies, *Haemostasis* (1986) **16**:386–416.

83. Vague P, Juhan-Vague I, Aillaud MF et al, Correlation between blood fibrinolytic activity, plasminogen activator inhibitor 1 level, plasma insulin level, and relative body weight in normal and obese subjects, *Metabolism* (1986) **35**:250–3.

84. Hamsten A, Karpe F, Bavenholm P, Silveria A, Interactions amongst insulin, lipoproteins and haemostatic function relevant to coronary heart disease, *J Intern Med* (1994) **236**(suppl 736):75–88.

85. Kjekshus J, Treating the diabetic patient with coronary disease, *Eur Heart J* (1996) **17**:1298–301.

86. Kwaan H, Changes in blood coagulation, platelet function and plasminogen–plasmin system in diabetes, *Diabetes* (1992) **41**(suppl 2):32–5.

87. Stubbs M, Jimenez A, Yamane M, Platelet hyper-reactivity in diabetics: relation to the time of onset of myocardial infarction, *JACC* (1990) **15**:119A.

88. Kannel WB, McGee DL, Diabetes and cardiovascular risk factors: the Framingham Study, *Circulation* (1979) **59**:8–13.

89. Ewing DJ, Campbell IW, Clarke BF, The natural history of diabetic autonomic neuropathy, *Q J Med* (1980) **493**:95–108.

90. Beere PA, Glagov S, Zarins CK, Retarding effect of lowered heart rate on coronary atherosclerosis, *Science* (1984) **226**:180–2.

91. Clarkson P, Celermajer DS, Donald AE et al, Impaired vascular reactivity in insulin dependent diabetes mellitus is related to disease, *J Am Coll Cardiol* (1996) **3**:573–9.

92. Jaffe AS, Spadaro JJ, Schechtman K, Roberts R, Geltman EM, Sobel BE, Increased congestive heart failure after myocardial infarction of modest extent in patients with diabetes mellitus, *Am Heart J* (1984) **108**:31–7.

93. Rodrigues B, McNeil JH, The diabetic heart: metabolic causes for the development of a cardiomyopathy, *Cardiovasc Res* (1992) **26**:913–22.

94. Granger C, Califf R, Young S et al, Outcome of patients with diabetes mellitus and acute myocardial infarction treated with thrombolytic agents, *J Am Coll Cardiol* (1993) **21**:290–5.

95. Davey G, McKeigue P, Insulin infusion in diabetic patients with acute myocardial infarction, *Br Med J* (1996) **313**:639–40.

96. Mjos OD, Effect of free fatty acids on myocardial infarction and oxygen consumption in tract dogs, *J Clin Invest* (1971) **50**:1386–9.

97. Malmberg K, Ryden L, Efendic S et al, Randomised trial of insulin–glucose infusion followed by subcutaenous insulin treatment in diabetic patients with acute myocardial infarction (DIGAMI study): effects on mortality at 1 year, *J Am Coll Cardiol* (1995) **26**:57–65.

98. Kjekshus J, Gilpin E, Cali G et al, Diabetic patients and beta-blockers after acute myocardial infarction. *Eur Heart J* (1990) **11**:43–50.

99. Gullestad L, Kjekshus J, Heart disease and diabetes melitus, *Tidsskr Nor Laegeforen* (1992); **112**:1016–19.

100. Norwegian Multicentre Study Group, Timolol-induced reduction in mortality and reinfarction in patients surviving acute myocardial infarction, *N Engl J Med* (1981) **304**:801–7.

101. Gundersent T, Kjeshus J, Timolol treatment after myocardial infarction in diabetic patients, *Diabetic Care* (1983); **6**:285–90.

102. Beta-blocker Heart Attack Trial Research Group. A randomised trial of propranolol in patients with acute myocardial infarction, Mortality results, *JAMA* (1982) **247**:1707–14.

103. Jonas M, Reicher-Reiss H, Boyko V et al. Usefulness of beta-blocker therapy in patients with non-insulin-dependent diabetes mellitus and coronary artery disease, *Am J Cardiol* (1996) **77**:1273–7.

104. Pyorala K, Pedersen TR, Kjekshus J et al, Cholesterol lowering with simvastatin improves prognosis of diabetic patients with coronary heart disease. A subgroup analysis of the Scandinavian Simvastatin Survival Study (4S). *Diabetes Care* (1997) **20**:614–20.

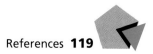

Chapter 4
Thromboembolism

Freek Verheugt

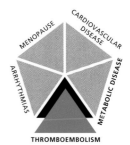

In many ways, the issue of thromboembolism provides the simplest treatment decisions for the clinician who is attempting to prevent coronary events. We will consider the therapeutic efficacy of antithrombotic therapy in the format shown in Table 4.1.

There is, of course, a vascular phase that precedes the platelet – that is, endothelial injury (plaque formation or hypertension) leads to exposure of a subendothelial vascular wall matrix, together with release of ADP and tissue thromboplastin. These events are dealt with elsewhere under lipid-lowering therapy and antihypertensive treatment.

Haemostatic phase	Primary prevention	Secondary prevention
Platelet phase	Aspirin	Aspirin
Coagulation phase		Heparin, warfarin
Fibrinolytic phase		Thrombolytics

Table 4.I Antithrombotic treatment strategies.

Furthermore, our focus is the long-term cardioprotective management of the patient at risk of coronary disease. Acute management with thrombolytics, aspirin and heparin is not our primary concern, although we must briefly review the current position of these treatments to place what follows in the wider context of thromboembolic risk.

First, however, we will give a brief but essential summary of the physiology of human haemostatic mechanisms.

■ PHYSIOLOGY OF HAEMOSTASIS

Endothelial cells play a central part in preventing vascular thrombosis. However, once endothelial integrity has been breached, there follows a cascade of events – release of ADP (a platelet aggregation factor) and tissue thromboplastin (tissue factor, a lipoprotein peptidase) – which leads to platelet activation by binding to factor VIII/vWF polymers and fibronectin, themselves released into the subendothelial matrix by endothelial cells. Platelet shape changes take place, the platelet adheres to the tissue matrix, and a release reaction ensues. Further ADP is secreted from platelet granules and a platelet phospholipase A_2 is activated. Thromboxane A_2 is subsequently generated, which leads to platelet aggregation. The further recruitment of platelets to the growing thrombus amplifies the release reaction.

Several other factors are produced during the release reaction, all of which will adversely effect the outcome of the patient at coronary risk:

- Serotonin – may cause coronary vasospasm.
- Platelet factor 4 – neutralizes the anticoagulant actions of circulating heparin.
- Platelet-derived growth factor – enhances smooth muscle cell proliferation and promotes atherogenesis.

Coagulation systems are divided into intrinsic and extrinsic. Their linked protease reactions convert proenzymes (inactive coagulation factors) into active enzymes.

The intrinsic system is activated after extravasation (in vitro, by contact with glass, kaolin and phospholipid), a process that involves factors XI and XII and a kininogen–prekallikrein complex. The extrinsic system relies on activation of factor VII to VIIa by tissue thromboplastin. These processes are summarized in Figure 4.1.

The fibrinolytic system limits thrombus formation and promotes clot lysis as the wound heals. Figure 4.2 shows the key steps. Plasminogen is converted to plasmin, a protease not normally found in the blood. Plasmin breaks fibrin down into fibrin degradation products. Plasmin generation is initiated by two plasminogen activators: tissue plasminogen activator (tPA) and single-chain urokinase-like plasminogen activator (scu-PA). tPA is inhibited in plasma by plasminogen activator inhibitors (PAI-1 or PAI-2), which are also derived from the endothelium. tPA and scu-PA bind selectively to fibrin on the thrombus surface. Plasminogen binds to this complex and is then converted to plasmin; hence the therapeutic thrombus specificity of the plasminogen activators. Alpha$_2$-antiplasmin is a natural inhibitor of plasmin.

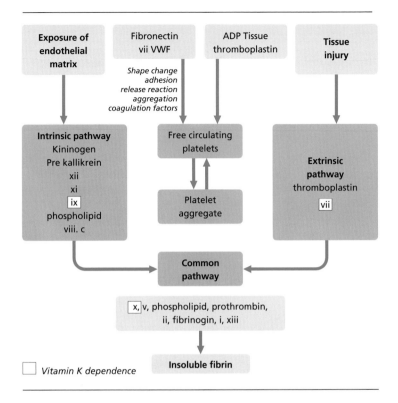

Figure 4.1 Haemostasis. Bold factors indicate vitamin K dependenc. Modified from Wintrobe et al, *Clinical Haematology*, 7th edn (Lea and Feibiger: Philadelphia 1974) 390, 420

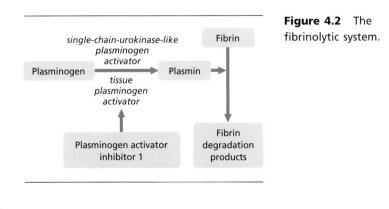

Figure 4.2 The fibrinolytic system.

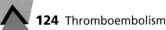

■ ACUTE MANAGEMENT

Thrombolytic therapy given within 12 h of onset of symptoms reduces mortality by about 25 per cent, irrespective of age, sex, blood pressure and site of myocardial infarction (MI) (anterior or inferior).[1] Aspirin 160 mg on admission and daily thereafter has an additive effect in reducing mortality and should be given to all patients as early as possible.

The debate has moved from *whether* thrombolysis works to *which* agent is most effective. The 'gridlock' in thrombolytic therapy – for example, ISIS-3[2] and GISSI-2[3] showed no difference in efficacy between tPA and streptokinase – seems to have been broken by the GUSTO (Global Utilisation of Streptokinase and tPA for Occluded Coronary Arteries) trial results.[4]

GUSTO enrolled 41 021 patients with an acute MI from over 1000 centres in 16 countries. Patients were randomized to receive one of four treatment regimens:

- Accelerated tPA (approximately 100 mg given over 90 min rather than the formerly recommended 3 h) + intravenous heparin
- tPA (1 mg/kg) + streptokinase 10^6 U + intravenous heparin
- Streptokinase 1.5×10^6 U + subcutaneous heparin
- Streptokinase 1.5×10^6 U + intravenous heparin

The accelerated tPA regimen reduced deaths from MI by 14 per cent compared with the other regimens, but was also associated with a higher risk of in-hospital stroke (1–2 per 1000; Table 4.2). Additionally, the efficacy of intravenous heparin when combined with tPA is, for some, now settled by GUSTO. The cost-effectiveness of tPA has been established.[5]

Some observers claim that a meta-analysis of all thrombolytic agents will put GUSTO into its proper context, and thus may eliminate the advantage of tPA. But the accelerated-dose regimen precludes combination of GUSTO with existing tPA data. Yet the question of acute treatment has now moved beyond even thrombolysis. A series of recent papers has suggested a superior cardioprotective efficacy of immediate percutaneous transluminal coronary angioplasty over both tPA[6] and streptokinase,[7] but in the much larger comparative GUSTO IIb trial this superiority can be questioned.[8] The ISIS-4 trial showed only modest benefit from an ACE inhibitor and no added

Treatment regimen	Mortality (%)	Disabling stroke (%)
Accelerated tPA + i.v. heparin	6.3	0.6
tPA + SK + i.v. heparin	7.0	0.6
SK + s.c. heparin	7.2	0.5
SK + i.v. heparin	7.4	0.5

tPA = tissue plasminogen activator
SK = streptokinase

Table 4.2 GUSTO: 30-day mortality and stroke rates.

benefit from nitrate or magnesium therapy above that of standard therapy for acute MI with or without streptokinase.[9] The proven efficacy of heparin with tPA will also provide added impetus to research into anticoagulants that are easier to administer and control, e.g. platelet activation inhibitors, thrombin inhibitors, such as the recombinant hirudins, and antibodies against the platelet fibrinogen receptor (glycoprotein IIb/IIIa receptor).[10]

■ CHRONIC MANAGEMENT

☐ Primary prevention

In patients without a history of vascular disease, there is no conclusive benefit of treatment with antiplatelet agents. The UK trial in British physicians[11] enrolled 5139 healthy male doctors over a 10-year period and openly randomized them 2:1 to 500 mg aspirin/day (or 330 mg enteric-coated aspirin) or to no aspirin. Although there was a 15 per cent reduction in mortality in the treated group, this did not achieve statistical significance (Figure 4.3). Moreover, no difference was found for non-fatal MI or stroke. Of most concern was a small excess of strokes in the treatment group.

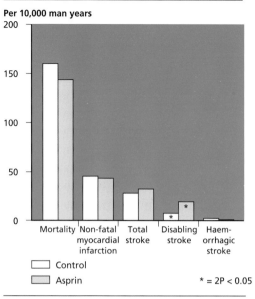

Figure 4.3 The UK physicians study

Per 10,000 man years

Control

Asprin

* = 2P < 0.05

The report of the US Physicians' Health Study[12] indicated that aspirin (325 mg aspirin on alternate days versus placebo in over 22 000 male subjects aged 40–84 years) reduced the rate of both fatal and non-fatal MI by 50 per cent although the total number of cardiovascular deaths in both treatment and control groups was the same (an excess of stroke and sudden death in the aspirin group) (Figure 4.4). This adverse 'trade-off' argues against primary prevention with aspirin. The US study also has serious drawbacks. The data and safety monitoring board stopped the trial at the halfway point and so further information on adverse events is limited. Moreover, extrapolation from a group of male physicians to the general population could be regarded as optimistic or pessimistic, depending on your point of view.[13]

In patients with unstable angina, aspirin (75 mg/day) will reduce the risk of an MI and death by about one-third (Figure 4.5).[14] This result substantiates data from three previous studies (Table 4.3).[15–17] Moreover, in patients with unstable angina

Chronic Management **127**

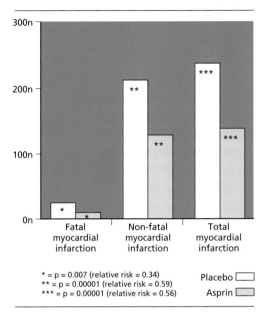

Figure 4.4 US physicians health study.

* = p = 0.007 (relative risk = 0.34)
** = p = 0.00001 (relative risk = 0.59)
*** = p = 0.00001 (relative risk = 0.56)

Placebo ☐
Asprin ▨

Trial	n	Aspirin dose	Endpoints that reached statistical significance in favour of aspirin
VA (1983)[15]	1266	324 mg/day	Combined MI + death; non-fatal MI
Canadian (1985)[16]	279	1.3 g/day	Cardiac death; total deaths
Montreal (1988)[17]	239	650 mg/day	MI
RISC (1990)[14]	796	75 mg/day	Combined MI + death

MI = myocardial infarction

Table 4.3 Aspirin in unstable angina.

Figure 4.5
RISC

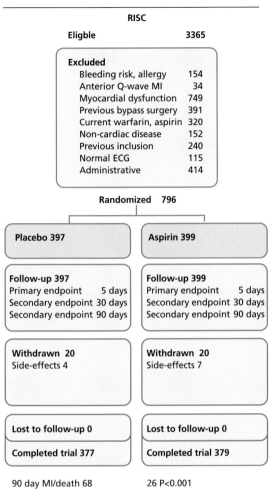

RISC

Eligble   3365

Excluded
Bleeding risk, allergy	154
Anterior Q-wave MI	34
Myocardial dysfunction	749
Previous bypass surgery	391
Current warfarin, aspirin	320
Non-cardiac disease	152
Previous inclusion	240
Normal ECG	115
Administrative	414

Randomized   796

Placebo 397

Aspirin 399

Follow-up 397
Primary endpoint   5 days
Secondary endpoint 30 days
Secondary endpoint 90 days

Follow-up 399
Primary endpoint   5 days
Secondary endpoint 30 days
Secondary endpoint 90 days

Withdrawn   20
Side-effects 4

Withdrawn   20
Side-effects 7

Lost to follow-up 0

Lost to follow-up 0

Completed trial 377

Completed trial 379

90 day MI/death 68   26 P<0.001

refractory to triple therapy with a nitrate, a calcium antagonist and a beta-blocker, an intravenous heparin infusion significantly reduces the frequency of angina episodes of silent ischaemia and total duration of ischaemia.[18] Possibly, subcutaneous low molecular weight heparin can achieve the same beneficial effect together with the advantages of prolonged ambulant use (Figure 4.6).[19]

Eligble   5137

Excluded

Bleeding risk	1023
Q-waves or bundle branch block (BBB)	717
Planned revascularization	156
Other cardiac diseases	116
Other severe diseases	218
Liver or kidney failure	120
Not recorded	54
Hypersensitivity	7
Compliance problems	762
Unwilling	458

Randomized   1506

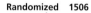

Placebo 760

Dalteparin 746

Follow-up 757
Primary endpoint   6 days
Secondary endpoints   30 days
Secondary endpoints   150 days

Follow-up 741
Primary endpoint   6 days
Secondary endpoints   30 days
Secondary endpoints   150 days

Withdrawn 274
Intravenous heparin or revascularization	132
Thrombolysis or Q-wave MI	36
Serious adverse event	14
Patient's request	63
Other	29

Withdrawn 268
Intravenous heparin or revascularization	97
Thrombolysis or Q-wave MI	23
Serious adverse event	17
Patient's request	84
Other	47

Lost to follow-up 3

Lost to follow-up 5

Completed trial 483

Completed trial 473

Death or MI   36 (4.8%)   13 (1.8%)
RR 0.37 (95% CI 0.20–0.68)

Figure 4.6   FRISC

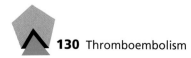

Antibodies against the platelet glycoprotein IIb/IIIa receptor given to patients undergoing high-risk coronary angioplasty have been shown to reduce the risk of MI and death by a third compared to aspirin.[20] Apparently, blockade of the final common pathway of platelet aggregation can protect patients better than inhibition of only the thromboxane pathway to aggregation.

☐ Secondary prevention

Antiplatelet agents

By 1980, six trials had investigated aspirin as a secondary preventive agent. A pooled analysis of these data[21] suggested that there was a clear benefit – a 10 per cent reduction in mortality and a 21 per cent reduction in reinfarction rate – for patients taking 1 g aspirin per day. The PARIS I[22] and PARIS II[23] studies confirmed this fall in reinfarction rate with this dose of aspirin.

In 1994, the Antiplatelet Trialists' Collaboration reported an analysis of 36 randomized trials on the role of aspirin in the prevention of both fatal and non-fatal MI and stroke in survivors of MI or in subjects with unstable angina or who had had transient ischaemic attacks of ischaemic strokes.[24] The main finding for secondary prevention of MI was a reduction of one-quarter in serious vascular events (13 per cent on aspirin versus 17 per cent in control groups) among 28 000 patients from 11 trials.

This meta-analysis was given added weight by the results of the ISIS-2 trial.[25] This study enrolled over 17 000 patients who were randomized to streptokinase and/or aspirin (160 mg/day enteric coated) was given for 5 weeks. Aspirin alone produced a 25 per cent odds reduction in vascular mortality, which, when it was given with streptokinase, increased to a 42 per cent fall in the same odds ratio (Table 4.4). ISIS-2 shows that aspirin 160 mg/day for 1 month would avoid 25 deaths and 10–15 reinfarctions and strokes per 1000 treated patients. One can add a further saving of 20 deaths over the subsequent 2–3 years with continuation of aspirin treatment if the results of the Antiplatelet Trialists' Collaboration are also taken into account.

Oral anticoagulants

The in-hospital mortality of patients following an acute MI, even with modern thrombolysis, is about 10 per cent. A further 10 per

	Streptokinase	No streptokinase	Aspirin	No aspirin	Streptokinase and aspirin	Neither
Vascular mortality	791	1029	804	1016	343	568
Non-fatal MI	238	202	156	284	77	123
Non-fatal stroke	37	41	27	51	13	27
Cerebral haemorrhage	7	0	5	2	5	0

Table 4.4 The ISIS-2 study.

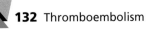

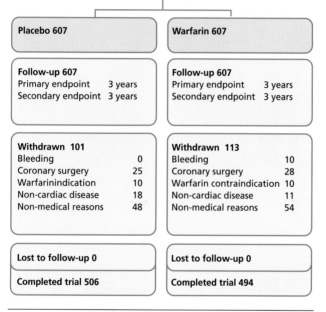

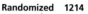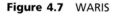

WARIS

Eligble	1918

Excluded

Death	16
Cancer	15
Indication to warfarin	156
Contraindication to warfarin	182
Administrative	65
Unwilling	270

Randomized 1214

Placebo 607	Warfarin 607

Follow-up 607	**Follow-up 607**
Primary endpoint 3 years	Primary endpoint 3 years
Secondary endpoint 3 years	Secondary endpoint 3 years

Withdrawn 101		**Withdrawn 113**	
Bleeding	0	Bleeding	10
Coronary surgery	25	Coronary surgery	28
Warfarinindication	10	Warfarin contraindication	10
Non-cardiac disease	18	Non-cardiac disease	11
Non-medical reasons	48	Non-medical reasons	54

Lost to follow-up 0	Lost to follow-up 0

Completed trial 506	Completed trial 494

Figure 4.7 WARIS

cent of patients die within 1 year of hospital discharge, beyond which mortality rates level out at 1–3 per cent per year. How might this high-risk 20 per cent be better managed? Might oral anticoagulants have a role?

The question of oral anticoagulant efficacy post-thrombolytic therapy has only been addressed in a relatively small angiographic trial[26] showing no benefit over aspirin or placebo.

However, an encouraging finding from one of the large thrombolysis trials does suggest that this group of drugs should receive further attention. In the AIMS trial,[27] after treatment with anistreplase or placebo plus heparin, warfarin was substituted for heparin and was continued for over 3 months in both groups. The in-hospital reduction in mortality (50.5 per cent) in the group receiving thrombolysis plus warfarin was the highest found in any thrombolytic trial.

In the Sixty Plus Trial,[28] 878 patients aged over 60 years (mean 67.6) who were receiving oral anticoagulants for up to 5 years after their index infarction were randomized to cessation or continuation of treatment. During 2 years of follow-up, mortality was reduced by 26 per cent and reinfarction rate fell by 55 per cent in the group continuing anticoagulant therapy. The frequency of intracranial haemorrhage was 1.6 per cent.

The Warfarin Reinfarction Study (Figure 4.7) compared warfarin and placebo for 37 months in 1214 patients (mean age 61.5 years) randomized at a mean of 27 days post-MI.[29] On warfarin, total mortality fell by 24 per cent, reinfarction rate fell by 34 per cent and stroke rates fell by 55 per cent. The frequency of intracranial haemorrhage was 0.8 per cent: thus, when compared with the Sixty Plus trial, risk seems related to age. The largest randomized placebo-controlled study of oral anticoagulants in modern cardiology was conducted in The Netherlands and showed, during a mean follow-up of 25 months, a non-significant (10 per cent) reduction of mortality and a 50 per cent reduction of reinfarction and 40 per cent reduction of total stroke.[30] About 25 per cent of patients had received thrombolysis prior to randomization in the trial. It should be noted that aspirin was not allowed in either WARIS or ASPECT, and a large trial directly comparing antiplatelet with oral anticoagulant therapy is urgently needed.

A new approach to oral platelet antagonism is the introduction of clopidogrel, the safe successor to ticlopidin, which induces neutropenia in a small percentage of patients. In the CAPRIE trial,[31] clopidogrel was compared with aspirin over a 2-year follow-up period in over 19 000 cardiovascular patients and found to reduce the endpoints death, myocardial (re)infarction and stroke by a mere 9 per cent. The over 6000 patients receiving clopidogrel or placebo after an MI did not benefit at all from the safe, but expensive, clopidogrel.

■ CONCLUSION

One can summarize the importance of treating (potential) thromboembolism associated with coronary artery disease (CAD) (Figure 4.8) as follows:

- Aspirin reduces deaths from MI in patients with unstable CAD by one-third, but is of no proven benefit in those without a history of vascular disease.

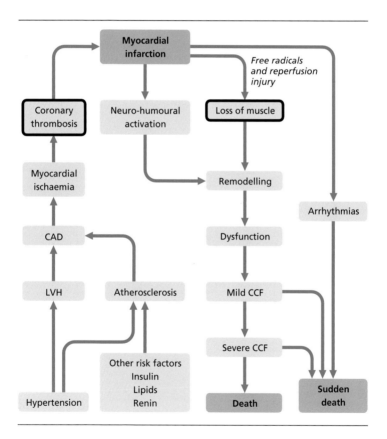

Figure 4.8   Interventions to limit thromboembolism in the ischaemic cycle.

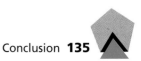

- Secondary prevention with aspirin in both the short and long term saves about 45 deaths per 1000 patients treated.
- Oral anticoagulants probably reduce mortality post-MI by about one-quarter, although this estimate requires formal confirmation in a randomized, controlled trial.

What of the future? The indications for antiplatelet therapy may be extended further. For example, in men with chronic stable angina, 325 mg aspirin on alternate days seems to produce an 86 per cent risk reduction for subsequent rates of MI.[32] This result was derived from a subgroup analysis of the US Physicians' Health Study and requires replication in a large clinical trial. The benefits of primary prevention with aspirin in women might also be a surprising finding when tested prospectively.[33] Studies in CAD, where oral anticoagulation is combined with low-dose aspirin, are underway.

Low-dose oral anticoagulation is currently under investigation in the Thrombosis Prevention Trial.[34] In this study, men at risk of coronary heart disease but who have not yet had an MI are being randomized to receive low-intensity oral anticoagulation with warfarin (INR 1.5) plus or minus aspirin.

Finally, prethrombotic status may predispose those who have cardiovascular risk factors to an increased frequency of coronary events. If such individuals can be identified – e.g. those with abnormal platelet function tests, high concentrations of PAI-1, protein C or protein S abnormalities, and other molecular markers of a predisposition to thrombosis – then targeted prophylaxis may be more effective than a global population-based approach.

References

1. Fibrinolytic Therapy Trialist's Collaborative Group, Indications for fibrinolytic therapy in suspected acute myocardial infarction: collaborative overview of early mortality and major morbidity results from all randomised trials of more than 1,000 patients, *Lancet* (1994) **343**:311–22.

2. ISIS-3 (Third International Study of Infarct Survival) Collaborative Group, A randomised comparison of streptokinase vs tissue plasminogen activator vs anistreplase and of aspirin plus heparin vs aspirin alone among 41 299 cases of suspected acute myocardial infarction: ISIS-3, *Lancet* (1992) **339**:753–70.

3. The international Study Group, In-hospital mortality and clinical course of 20,891 patients with suspected acute myocardial

infarction randomised between alteplase and streptokinase with or without heparin, *Lancet* (1990) **336**:71–5.

4. GUSTO Investigators, An international randomized trial comparing four thrombolytic strategies for acute myocardial infarction, *N Engl J Med* (1993) **329**:673–82.

5. Mark DB, Hlatky MA, Califf RM et al, Cost-effectiveness of thrombolytic therapy with tissue plasminogen activator as compared to streptokinase for acute myocardial infarction, *N Engl J Med* (1995) **332**:1418–24.

6. Grines CL, Browne KF, Marco J et al, A comparison of immediate angioplasty with thrombolytic therapy for acute myocardial infarction, *N Engl J Med* (1993) **328**:673–9.

7. Zijlstra F, De Boer MJ, Hoorntje JCA, Reiffers S, Reiber JHC, Suryapranata H, A comparison of immediate angioplasty with intravenous streptokinase in acute myocardial infarction, *N Engl J Med* (1993) **328**:680–4.

8. Verheugt FWA, Primary angioplasty for acute myocardial infarction: is the balloon half full or half empty? *Lancet* (1996) **347**:1276–7.

9. Four International Study of Infarct Survival Collaborative Group, ISIS-4: a randomised factorial trial assessing early oral captopril, oral mononitrate, and intravenous magnesium sulphate in 58 050 patients with suspected acute mycardial infarction, *Lancet* (1995) **345**:669–85.

10. Lefkovits J, Plow EF, Topol EJ, Platelet glycoprotein IIb/IIIa receptors in cardiovascular medicine, *N Engl J Med* (1995) **332**:1553–9.

11. Peto R, Gray R, Collins R et al, Randomised trial of prophylactic daily aspirin in British male doctors, *Br Med J* (1988) **296**:313–16.

12. Steering Committee of the Physicians Health Study Research Group, Final report on the aspirin component of the ongoing Physicians' Health Study, *N Engl J Med* (1989) **321**:129–35.

13. Horton RC, Kendall MJ, Aspirin in the next decade, *J Clin Pharm Ther* (1989) **14**:249–61.

14. RISC Group, Risk of myocardial infarction and death during treatment with low dose aspirin and intravenous heparin in men with unstable coronary artery disease, *Lancet* (1990) **336**:827–30.

15. Lewis HD Jr, Davi JW, Archibald DG et al, Protective effects of aspirin against acute myocardial infarction and death in men with unstable angina: results of a Veterans Administration Cooperative Study, *N Engl J Med* (1983) **309**:396–403.

16. Cairns JA, Gent M, Singer et al, Aspirin, sulfinpyrazone or both in unstable angina pectoris: results of a Canadian multicenter trial, *N Engl J Med* (1985) **311**:1369–75.

17. Théroux P, Ouimet H, McCans J et al, Aspirin, heparin, or both to treat acute unstable angina, *N Engl J Med* (1988) **319**:1105–111.

18. Neriserneri GG, Gensini GF, Poggesi L et al, Effect of heparin, aspirin, or alteplase in reduction of myocardial ischemia in refractory unstable angina, *Lancet* (1990) **335**:615–18.

19. FRISC Study Group, Low-molecular-weight heparin using instability in coronary artery disease, *Lancet* (1996) **347**:561–8.

20. The EPIC Investigation, Use of a monoclonal antibody directed against the platelet glycoprotein IIb/IIIa receptor in high-risk coronary angioplasty, *N Engl J Med* (1994) **330**:956–61.

21. Editorial, Aspirin after myocardial infarction, *Lancet* (1980) **i**:1172–3.

22. The Persantine–Aspirin Reinfarction Study Group, Persantine and aspirin in coronary heart disease, *Circulation* (1980) **62**:449–61.

23. Klimt C, Knatterud L, Stamler J, Meier P, Persantine–Aspirin Reinfarction Study. Part II. Secondary coronary prevention with persantine and aspirin, *J Am Coll Cardiol* (1986) **7**:251–69.

24. Antiplatelet Trialists' Collaboration, Collaborative overview of randomised trials of antiplatelet therapy I: prevention of death, myocardial infarction, and stroke by prolonged antiplatelet therapy in various categories of patients, *Br Med J* (1994) **308**:81–106.

25. ISIS-2 (Second International Study of Infarct Survival) Collaborative Group, Randomised trial of intravenous streptokinase, oral aspirin, both, or neither among 17,187 cases of suspected acute myocardial infarction: ISIS-2, *Lancet* (1988) **ii**:349–60.

26. Meijer A, Verheugt FWA, Werter CJPJ, Lie KI, Van der Pol JMJ, Van Eenige MJ, Aspirin versus coumadin in the prevention of reocclusion and recurrent ischemia after successful thrombolysis: a prospective placebo-controlled angiographic study: results of the APRICOT Study, *Circulation* (1993) **87**:1524–30.

27. AIMS Trial Study Group, Effect of intravenous APSAC on mortality after acute myocardial infarction: preliminary report of a placebo-controlled clinical trial, *Lancet* (1988) **i**:545–9.

28. Sixty Plus Reinfarction Study Research Group, A double-blind trial to assess long-term oral anticoagulant therapy in elderly patients after myocardial infarction, *Lancet* (1980) **ii**:989–94.

29. Smith P, Arnesen H, Holme I, The effect of warfarin on mortality and reinfarction after myocardial infarctions, *N Engl J Med* (1990) **323**:147–52.

30. Anticoagulants in the Secondary Prevention of Events in Coronary Thrombosis (ASPECT) Research Group, Effect of long-term oral anticoagulant treatment on mortality and cardiovascular morbidity after myocardial infarction, *Lancet* (1994) **343**:499–503.

31. CAPRIE Steering Committee, A randomised, blinded, trial of clopidogrel versus aspirin in patients at risk of ischaemic events (CAPRIE), *Lancet* (1996) **349**:1329–39.

32. Ridker PM, Manson JAE, Gaziano JM, Buring JE, Hennekens CH, Low-dose aspirin for chronic stable angina: a randomized, placebo-controlled clinical trial, *Arch Intern Med* (1991) **114**:835–9.

33. Manson JE, Stampfer MJ, Colditz GA et al, A prospective study of aspirin use and primary prevention of cardiovascular disease in women, *JAMA* (1991) **266**:521–7.

34. Meade TW, Roderick PJ, Brennan PJ, Wilkes HC, Kelleher CC, Extra-cranial bleeding and other symptoms due to low dose aspirin and low intensity oral anticoagulation, *Thromb Haemost* (1992) **68**:1–6.

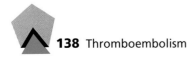

Chapter 5
The drug treatment of arrhythmias

Ronald Campbell

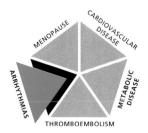

■ INTRODUCTION

Cardiac arrhythmias constitute a common and feared complication of ischaemic heart disease, They may be associated with all forms of ischaemic heart disease from coronary artery spasm, as in Prinzmetal's variant angina, which has a well-recognized arrhythmic risk,[1] through stable and unstable angina, and from acute infarction to the post-acute recovery phase. It is in the earliest minutes of acute myocardial (AMI) infarction that the greatest risk is seen.[2] It is widely held that the early 35–40 per cent mortality of acute coronary artery occlusion is due to ventricular fibrillation (VF).

There is no evidence that arrhythmias are involved in the genesis of ischaemic heart disease but they certainly can be detrimental to the course of the illness. Arrhythmias may produce haemodynamic embarrassment, may jeopardize myocardial perfusion, or, worst of all, may kill directly. The importance of the arrhythmic complications of ischaemic heart disease is becoming more obvious with the spectacular improvements in the management of ischaemia and in the salvage of jeopardized myocardium.

There is no shortage of drugs which have antiarrhythmic actions, but results of most large-scale randomized controlled studies of antiarrhythmic therapies in ischaemic disease have proved disappointing[3–19] (Tables 5.1 and 5.2). Part of the problem may lie in the inability of most antiarrhythmic drugs to prevent VF. Many are effective in controlling ventricular ectopic beats and ventricular tachycardia, but the mechanism of these arrhythmias is fundamentally different from that of VF.

■ ANTIARRHYTHMIC THERAPY IN ACUTE-PHASE MYOCARDIAL INFARCTION

The electrophysiological consequences of acute coronary occlusion have been extensively investigated. Much work has been performed in animals, as it is difficult to acquire human data in the earliest moments of the event. Paramedic rescue squads have begun to provide such information, and all evidence would suggest that there is a high initial risk of VF which declines

Author	Year	n	Agent	Analysis period	Total mortality (%)	Arrhythmic or sudden death (or surrogate) (%)	Comment
Snow[3]	1965	45	Propranolol	28 days	16 $p < 0.025$	7 NS	
		46	Placebo		37	13	
Koster and Dunning[4]	1985	2987	Lidocaine	15–60 min	0.6 NS	0.06 $p < 0.01$	Intramuscular dosing
		3037	Placebo		0.7	0.4	
Campbell et al[5]	1983	278	Tocainide	48 h	2	4	Acute intravenous study
		281	Placebo		NS 3	NS 2	
ISIS – I[6]	1986	8037	Atenolol	3 days	3.9 $p < 0.04$	2.2 $p < 0.05$	
		7990	Control		4.6	2.6	

Table 5.1 Selected comparative controlled studies of prophylactic antiarrhythmic therapy in acute phase myocardial infarction.

Author	Year	n	Agent	Analysis period	Total mortality (%)	Arrhythmic or sudden death (or surrogate) (%)	Comment
Chamberlain et al[7]	1980	181 163	Mexiletine Placebo	3 months	13 NS 12	–	
IMPACT[8]	1984	317 313	Mexiletine (LA) Placebo	9 months	8 NS 5	2 NS 1	First study to show significant adverse impact of treatment. Stopped prematurely
CAST I[9]	1989	730 725	Flecainide Encainide } Placebo	10 months	8 8 $p < 0.0003$ 3	5 $p < 0.0008$ 1	Stopped prematurely
CAST II[10]	1992	665 660	Moricizine Placebo	14 days	3 $p < 0.01$ 0.5	1.4 0.5	Enrolled 'responders' to moricizine. Stopped prematurely
Julian et al[11]	1982	873 583	Sotalol Placebo	1 year	7.3 NS 8.9	2.9 NS 2.4	Sudden death <1 h from symptoms
Burkart et al (BASIS)[12]	1990	98 100 114	Amiodarone 'Conventional' Placebo	1 year	5 $p < 0.05$ 10 13	–	
Ceremuzynski[13]	1993	305 308	Amiodarone Placebo	1 year	7 NS 11	–	Enrolled those not eligible for beta-blockers. Cardiac mortaility reduced by amiodarone

	Year	n	Drug	Duration	Total mortality	Arrhythmic death	Comments
Doval et al[14]	1994	260	Amiodarone	2 years	34 $p < 0.024$	12 NS	
		256	Placebo		41	15	
Singh et al[15]	1995	336	Amiodarone	2 years	31 NS	15 NS	
		338	Placebo		29	19	
Cairns et al (CAMIAT)[16]	1997	606	Amiodarone	2 years	6 NS	2 $p < 0.016$	
		596	Placebo		8	5	
Julian et al (EMIAT)[17]	1997	743	Amiodarone	2 years	14 NS	6 $p < 0.05$	
		743	Placebo		14	8	
Waldo et al[18]	1996	1549	d-Sotalol	148 days	5 $p < 0.006$	4 $p < 0.008$	Increased 'total mortality' and 'presumed arrhythmic death'
		1572	Placebo		3	2	
DAVIT II[19]	1990	878	Verapamil	18 months	11 NS	6 NS	
		897	Placebo		14	7	

LA = long acting
NS = not significant.

Table 5.2 Selected comparative controlled studies of prophylactic antiarrhythmic therapy in post MI patients and in ischeamic heart failure.

exponentially with time.[20] The risk of VF is relatively low 12 h after the acute event.[2] This corresponds to a time when all myocardium expected to die will have ceased to have electrical activity. Acute myocardial ischaemia shortens local refractoriness and creates conditions of regional inhomogeneity.[21] This effect of ischaemia has been shown clinically by increased QT dispersion recorded by conventional electrocardiography.[22]

Analysis of incidents of early VF shows their near-universal provocation by an R-on-T ventricular ectopic beat.[23] It was natural, therefore, that such beats, and R-on-T beats in particular, might be a target for drug intervention in the expectation that VF rates could be reduced. Many different agents have been studied.

☐ Class I drugs – sodium channel blockers

Several studies have examined lignocaine given parenterally, but it was not until the study of Koster and Dunning[4] that a robust scientific answer on the value of lignocaine was forthcoming. These investigators enrolled patients seen out of hospital by paramedics. Intramuscular lignocaine was given in a double-blind manner. Patients receiving the active therapy had significantly fewer incidents of primary VF than their placebo-treated counterparts, but those receiving lignocaine had a significant increase of heart block and asystole which almost exactly counterbalanced the benefit in VF protection. The evidence was that VF could be prevented in part by lignocaine therapy but that the risks of therapy outweighed its benefit. Moreover, no overall mortality benefit was seen. Results using other sodium channel blocking drugs acutely are no more encouraging, with none showing net benefit. In a study of tocainide, a close structural analogue of lignocaine, no anti-VF effect was seen.[5]

☐ Class II drugs – beta-blockers

Beta-blockers have been thoroughly investigated in acute-phase MI and have been shown to offer improved prognosis.[6] There has been only minimal evidence, however, that the benefit was due to an arrhythmic effect.

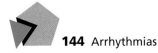

144 Arrhythmias

In 1965, Snow reported a significant improvement in mortality associated with propranolol therapy.[3] ECG monitoring was not available, precluding identification of the mechanism of benefit. This study was relatively small. Subsequent studies focused on the use of beta-blockers to influence infarction size and total mortality, and to control chest pain. The results identified a role for beta-blockade in acute-phase MI, with some hints that an anti-VF effect might also be present. In the ISIS-I study, atenolol was given intravenously in the acute-phase MI and was associated with a significant reduction of primary VF.[6]

☐ Effects of reperfusion

Acute-phase MI is now aggressively treated by thrombolytic agents. These are not conventionally considered antiarrhythmic drugs, but by re-establishing a blood supply to jeopardized myocardium, they bring electrophysiological benefits.[24] Subsequent to reperfusion, the incidence of VF is reduced.[25] The act of reperfusion, however, may provoke VF in itself.[26] Reperfusional VF is a common problem in animal models, and it was feared that it would prove similarly problematic in humans. Happily, the evidence is to the contrary. Reperfusional VF is probably related to time from onset of symptoms and to the speed and extent of myocardial reperfusion.

■ ANTIARRHYTHMIC THERAPY IN LATE-PHASE MYOCARDIAL INFARCTION

Ventricular arrhythmias are common in survivors of the hospital phase of MI. Their presence has been investigated as a potential indicator of a poor prognosis. In the 1980s post-MI ventricular ectopic beat rates that exceeded more than 10 beats/h were linked with an increased risk of death.[27] Evidence at that time was insufficiently precise to determine the ways in which patients died, but death was not restricted to arrhythmic forms. Subsequent investigations have shown that the sensitivity and specificity of ventricular ectopic beats to define prognosis is relatively modest.[28] In multivariate analysis, however, ventricular ectopic beat frequency remains an independent predictor[28] and, until recently, it was plausible to imagine that suppression of ventricular ectopic beats might be rewarded by an improved prognosis.

☐ Post MI class I drugs – early studies (pre-CAST[9])

Between 1970 and 1989, many studies examined the role of antiarrhythmic drugs in improving prognosis for survivors of AMI. Most, by modern standards, would be judged as inadequate. These studies enrolled high-risk survivors of infarction but, curiously, in very few studies were ventricular ectopic beats a specified inclusion criterion. The results of using drugs such as procainamide, phenytoin, quinidine and mexiletine were disappointing.[29] In several, mortality was higher for those patients receiving the active antiarrhythmic drug than in those receiving placebo therapy[7,8] (Tables 5.1 and 5.2). Yet 24–h ECG recordings suggested that the drugs reduced ventricular ectopic beat frequency. An explanation advanced for the lack of impact on mortality was that the agents used were inadequately powerful. It was considered not enough to reduce ventricular ectopic beats; they had to be abolished. This was not an unreasonable concept, given the evidence that it required only one ectopic beat to trigger VF.

☐ Post MI class I drugs – CAST and post-CAST

The introduction of the class 1c antiarrhythmic drugs flecainide and encainide provided a tool to test the effects of more profound ventricular ectopic beat suppression than had been possible with older drugs. The Cardiac Arrhythmia Suppression Trial[9] enrolled patients with manifest ventricular ectopic beats and sought to show that near-complete suppression would be rewarded with an improved prognosis. The study was prematurely terminated when a significant excess mortality was seen in patients receiving flecainide and encainide.[9] Even now, almost 10 years after that study, its results have far-reaching consequences. Many workers have sought to explain the unexpected outcome. Of the many points advanced, perhaps the most important is the very low

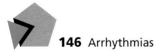

mortality (3 per cent) in patients who received placebo therapy. With such a low risk of death it was probably unreasonable to expect that any improvement would be identified. Indeed, with such a low placebo mortality, the situation was biased to expose any shortcomings of the therapy, as proved to be the case. The actual mechanism of the increased mortality is unknown. Most workers suggest that arrhythmogenesis, particularly the creation of torsade des pointes, was responsible. Despite the increased rate of sudden, presumptively arrhythmic death (Table 5.2), there is no firm evidence for this. It is equally plausible that patients who, for instance, developed new ischaemic events were haemodynamically disadvantaged by being on the active antiarrhythmic drug. The Cardiac Arrhythmia Suppression Trial arm involving moricizine was continued as CAST II, but this too was terminated by an increased mortality related to the antiarrhythmic agent.[10]

These results appear to preclude any general role for class 1 antiarrhythmic drugs in improving prognosis for unselected patients post-MI.

☐ Post-MI class II drugs

Beta-blockers given to post-MI patients improve prognosis.[6] The mechanism of benefit is not well understood, as these drugs potentially offer antiarrhythmic and anti-ischaemic actions. One small study has linked beta-blocker effects with suppression of ventricular arrhythmias,[30] but this falls well short of substantiating that beta-blockers prevent VF.

In a study of sotalol, arguably a beta-blocker with special antiarrhythmic potential, total mortality was not significantly reduced, although the risk reduction was similar to that observed in larger investigations.[11] Sotalol-treated patients in that study had a marginally higher mortality in the first week of treatment than did their placebo-treated counterparts. This may merely be a chance observation but it raises concerns of early detriment with this agent.

☐ Post-MI class III drugs

The most recent studies of antiarrhythmic drug use in post-MI patients have involved amiodarone. This powerful antiarrhythmic drug can probably act against VF. In the first reported study, the Basel Antiarrhythmic Study of Infarct Survival (BASIS), patients with ventricular ectopic beats post-MI who received amiodarone fared statistically significantly better than those patients given no therapy and better than those given individualized conventional antiarrhythmic therapy.[12] In a subsequent analysis of this study, it was suggested that the benefit accrued only to those with good left ventricular function and that the outcome for those with ejection fractions of less than 30 per cent was uninfluenced by the prescription of amiodarone.[31] Subsequently in a Polish study, post-MI sudden death rates for those on amiodarone were significantly reduced and there was a trend favouring a reduction in total mortality.[13] Patients in this study were recruited according to a variety of high-risk features, including the presence of frequent ventricular ectopic beats.

Two further studies have focused principally upon patients with heart failure, but many were post-MI. In the South American GESICA study, mortality was significantly reduced and there was a trend for reduction in sudden death rates.[14] Subgroup analysis suggested that the benefits accrued principally to those with non-ischaemic reasons for heart failure. In the Veterans Administration Study, no mortality benefit was identified.[15] In this study, the majority of patients had an ischaemic background.

The most up-to-date information comes from the European and Canadian Amiodarone in Infarction Trials (CAMIAT[16] and EMIAT[17]).

These studies together recruited more than 2600 patients and were designed as the definitive evaluations of amiodarone in post-MI patients. EMIAT's primary endpoint was total (all-cause) mortality, while CAMIAT's was a composite of resuscitated VF or arrhythmic death.

EMIAT enrolled MI survivors with left ventricular ejection fractions of ≤ 40 per cent. Manifest arrhythmias were not a prerequisite for inclusion. There were 103 deaths in those randomized to amiodarone ($n = 743$) and 102 in the placebo group ($n = 743$). Total mortality was clearly uninfluenced by amiodarone. Although controversial, detailed validation of cause of death allowed examination of a secondary endpoint – arrhythmic death. This was reduced from 50 such events in the placebo group (7 per cent) to 33 events in those randomized to amiodarone (4 per cent, $P = 0.05$). It is as yet unexplained why this possible antiarrhythmic effect was not reflected in the total mortality analysis. Non-arrhythmic cardiac deaths and non-cardiac deaths were increased in those in the amiodarone group. Three of the latter deaths were due to pulmonary fibrosis but, with the exception of thyroid and liver disorders, unwanted effects were of similar frequency in the placebo group. No patient, whether allocated to placebo or amiodorone, had documented torsade de pointes. The authors appropriately commented that the findings did not support the systematic prophylactic use of amiodarone in all patients with depressed left ventricular function after MI.

The CAMIAT findings are almost identical, yet they have been given a different profile in that the primary endpoint (resuscitated VF or arrhythmic death) was significantly reduced in amiodarone-allocated patients (6 per cent placebo, 3 per cent amiodarone; $P = 0.016$). The secondary endpoint of total (all-cause) mortality was unchanged by treatment allocation (57 of 606 amiodarone patients (9 per cent) versus 68 of 596 placebo patients (11 per cent)). Unlike in EMIAT, however, there was no evidence of increased non-arrhythmic cardiac deaths or of non-cardiac deaths. A further important feature is that patients included in CAMIAT had their qualifying MI complicated by ventricular ectopic beats ($\geq$ 10/h or at least one run of ventricular tachycardia) rather than by left ventricular dysfunction. The CAMIAT authors suggest that 'treatment decisions for individual survivors should require an assessment of their baseline risk factors and judgements based on the synthesis of our findings with those of related trials'.

EMIAT and CAMIAT have not clarified the situation regarding amiodarone use post-MI. The strongest evidence is that amiodarone has a tangible and potentially valuable antiarrhythmic effect against lethal arrhythmias but, as yet, patient selection is not well refined and there are important concerns regarding the potential for increased non-arrhythmic and non-cardiac deaths when using this agent.

The dextro isomer of sotalol has been investigated in post-MI patients who had left ventricular dysfunction or whose MI was complicated by features of heart failure.[18] This study was prematurely terminated with a statistically significant increased mortality in d-sotalol patients (5.0 per cent versus 3.1 per cent, $P < 0.05$). Presumed arrhythmic death was also significantly increased (Table 5.2).

☐ Post-MI class IV drugs

Diltiazem has been studied in post-MI patients.[19] Although some 'benefits' were reported in those with non-Q-wave infarction, total mortality and sudden death rates were not reduced by this therapy.

■ SPECIFIC POST-MI PATIENTS

Most of the studies so far described have enrolled post-MI patients who, at best, are stratified by ejection fraction but who are not defined as being at particularly high risk of sudden, presumptively or definitely, *arrhythmic* death. Prevention of post-MI VF is not the only application for antiarrhythmic therapy. Patients who show sustained monomorphic ventricular tachycardia post-MI are at high risk of recurrences.[32] These ventricular tachyarrhythmias are dangerous, as their rate is often rapid and degeneration to VF may occur. Affected patients have a poor prognosis. Monomorphic ventricular tachycardia can usually be reliably provoked and terminated by programmed stimulation. The arrhythmia mechanism is probably macro-re-entry. Antiarrhythmic drugs can be tested in an electrophysiological (EP) study. Patients in whom they prevent the reinitiation of the native ventricular tachycardia have a good prognosis.[33] Whether to obtain the good prognosis requires the continued prescription of the antiarrhythmic drug or whether it is the drug suppressibility of the arrhythmia that is the prognostic marker remains controversial. For the present, most would prescribe chronic antiarrhythmic therapy as identified by the EP study.

In patients in whom no effective antiarrhythmic drug can be found by EP testing, 'blind' amiodarone therapy offers some benefit with reduced recurrence rates and a possibly improved prognosis. In this context, however, there is a growing role for the implantable cardioverter defibrillator.[34] These devices can and do prevent arrhythmic death.[35,36] Their optimal utilization is in those patients who are identified as being at particular risk of lethal arrhythmias. More work has to be done to stratify infarction survivors in this regard, but early studies look

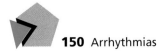

promising. In studies which have compared 'blind' amiodarone with the use of the ICD, ICD figures are superior. The publication of the first randomized comparative study of the ICD versus 'conventional' therapy in patients with infarction who suffered a late cardiac arrest revealed a statistically significant superiority of the ICD in terms of survival (86 per cent ICD survival versus 65 per cent 'conventional' therapy).[36] Were it not for the specialist nature of the devices and their not inconsiderable cost, they would have a wider application than is currently the case.

■ ATRIAL FIBRILLATION

Atrial fibrillation is an important arrhythmia in whatever pathological context it occurs. Cardiac ischaemia is no exception.

□ Acute myocardial infarction

Atrial fibrillation is not promoted by either stable or unstable angina. When it complicates AMI, it reflects either atrial infarction and/or a major ventricular infarction with significant cardiac decompensation. Given these associations, atrial fibrillation obviously has prognostic importance. Management is to deal speedily with the haemodynamic consequences of the arrhythmia. DC cardioversion to sinus rhythm might at first seem the best option, but as the initial precipitating factors will still be present, high relapse rates should be expected. Conventional approaches to ventricular rate control would involve digoxin with or without the adjunctive action of a calcium entry agent or a beta-blocker. Parenteral amiodarone may be a useful alternative.[37] This is very effective in restoring sinus rhythm and, in the event of atrial fibrillation not responding, it will slow the ventricular response by its effect on the AV node. Few patients remain in atrial fibrillation beyond the first 48 h of infarction, but warfarin anticoagulation is advisable in all patients, as infarction is associated with a thrombotic state, and the risk of thromboembolism is appreciable.

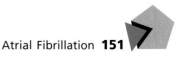

☐ Post-CABG

Atrial fibrillation is an important complication of coronary artery disease treated by coronary artery bypass grafting (CABG). Up to 25 per cent of operated patients are affected.[38] Events are usually short-lived (2–3 days) and occur usually on postoperative days 2 or 3. Preoperative withdrawal of beta-blockers has been linked with the development of the arrhythmia, and with more aggressive approaches to the use and maintenance of beta-blockade this complication is less frequent. Many antiarrhythmic drugs have been tested for their ability to prevent postoperative atrial fibrillation but most are inappropriate for clinical use. A beta-blocker, given parenterally if necessary, is the best first-line approach.[39] If there is haemodynamic concern, parenteral amiodarone for 24–48 h is recommended. As with post-MI patients, warfarin anticoagulation should be given. There is no evidence that postoperative atrial fibrillation carries any late prognostic significance.

■ RISK PREDICTION

Arrhythmias are only one mechanism of death for patients with coronary heart disease. Much effort has been expended on identification of predictors of total mortality, particularly in post-MI patients. Much less has been done to identify risk factors for sudden, presumptively arrhythmic death and almost nothing is known of such risk factors in those with angina rather than infarction. These are serious deficiencies. Were it possible to identify those at particular risk of arrhythmic death, protective antiarrhythmic strategies could be better profiled. Table 5.3 lists the features that have been shown to be predictive of late sustained ventricular tachycardia, of sudden, presumptively arrhythmic death and of total mortality in post-MI patients. None are particularly impressive in terms of sensitivity or specificity. Not surprisingly, prediction of total mortality can be improved by combining a variety of risk factors. Nonetheless, we are still a long way from clinically useful individualized risk prediction.

Sustained VT	Sudden presumptive arrhythmia death	Total mortality
Signal-averaged late potentials	QT dispersion EP testing	Ejection fraction Effort testing
EP testing		Cardiothoracic ratio Ventricular ectopic beats on Holter Heart rate variability Baroreflex sensitivity QT interval Troponin T Fibrinogen Lipids

Table 5.3 Post-MI predictors of sustained VT, sudden presumptive arrhythmic death and total mortality

■ CONCLUSIONS

Any cardiac disease may reduce the threshold for lethal arrhythmias. The goal of clinical management must be to prevent myocardial damage and to remove regional abnormalities of perfusion, contraction and electrophysiology. Antiarrhythmic drugs are a crude intervention and most have not been developed as anti-VF agents. They operate best against ventricular ectopic beats, which probably arise by triggered automaticity. Beta-blockers and amiodarone probably do have actions against VF and they have produced the most promising results in terms of prognosis. It remains the case however, that once VF starts, no currently available drug is likely to encourage its self-termination. In that circumstance, only external or internal cardioversion can save the patient's life.

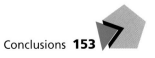

References

1. Guazzi M, Fiorentini C, Polese A et al, Continuous electrocardiographic recording in Prinzmetal's variant angina pectoris. A report of four cases, *Br Heart J* (1970) **32** (5):611–16.

2. Adgey AAJ, Allen JD, Geddes JS et al, Acute phase of myocardial infarction, *Lancet* (1971) **2**:501-4.

3. Snow PJD, Effect of propranolol in myocardial infarction, *Lancet* (1965) **2**:551–3.

4. Koster RW, Dunning AJ, Intramuscular lidocaine for prevention of lethal arrhythmias in the prehospitalisation phase of acute myocardial infarction, *N Engl J Med* (1985) **313**:1105–10.

5. Campbell RWF, Hutton I, Elton RA et al, Prophylaxis of primary ventricular fibrillation with tocainide in acute myocardial infarction, *Br Heart J* (1983) **49**:557–63.

6. ISIS-I. First International Study of Infarct Survival Collaborative Group, Randomised trial of intravenous atenolol among 16,027 cases of suspected acute myocardial infarction, *Lancet* (1986) **2**:57–66.

7. Chamberlain DA, Jewitt DE, Julian DG et al, Oral mexiletine in high-risk patients after myocardial infarction, *Lancet* (1980) **ii**:1324–7.

8. IMPACT Research Group, International mexiletine and placebo antiarrhythmic coronary trial: l. Report on arrhythmia and other findings, *J Am Coll Cardiol* (1984) **4** (6):1148–63.

9. The Cardiac Arrhythmia Suppression Trial Investigators, Preliminary report: effect of encainide and flecainide on mortality in a randomized trial of arrhythmia suppression after myocardial infarction, *N Engl J Med* (1989) **321**:406–12.

10. The Cardiac Arrhythmia Suppression Trial II Investigators, Effect of the antiarrhythmic agent moricizine on survival after myocardial infarction, *N Engl J Med* (1992) **327**:227–33.

11. Julian DG, Jackson FS, Prescott RJ et al, Controlled trial of sotalol for one year after myocardial infarction, *Lancet* (1982) **i**:1142–7.

12. Burkart FF, Pfisterer M, Kiowski W et al, Effect of antiarrhythmic therapy on mortality in survivors of myocardial infarction with asymptomatic complex ventricular arrhythmias: Basel Antiarrhythmic Study of Infarct Survival (BASIS), *J Am Coll Cardiol* (1990) **16** (7):1711–18.

13. Ceremuzynski L, Secondary prevention after myocardial infarction with Class III antiarrhythmic drugs, *Am J Cardiol* (1993) **72** (16):F82–6.

14. Doval HC, Nul DR, Grancelli HO et al, Randomised trial of low-dose amiodarone in severe congestive heart failure, *Lancet* (1994) **344**:493–8.

15. Singh SN, Fletcher RD, Fisher SG et al, Amiodarone in patients with congestive heart failure and asymptomatic ventricular arrhythmia. Survival Trial of Antiarrhythmic Therapy in Congestive Heart Failure, *N Engl J Med* (1995) **333** (2):77–82.

16. Cairns JA, Connolly SJ, Roberts R et al, Canadian Amiodarone Myocardial Infarction Arrhythmia Trial (CAMIAT): rationale and protocol, *Am J Cardiol* (1993) **72** (16):87F–94F.

17. Julian DG, Camm AJ, Frangin G et al, for the European Myocardial Infarct Amiodarone Trial Investigators, Randomised trial of effect of amiodarone on mortality in patients with left-ventricular dysfunction after recent myocardial infarction: EMIAT, *Lancet* (1997) **349** (9053):667–74.

18. Waldo AL, Camm AJ, deRuyter H et al, for the SWORD investigators, Effect of d-sotalol on mortality in patients with left ventricular dysfunction after recent and remote myocardial infarction, *Lancet* (1996) **348**:7–12.

19. Anonymous, Effect of verapamil on mortality and major events after acute myocardial infarction (the Danish Verapamil Infarction Trial II – DAVIT II), *Am J Cardiol* (1990) **66** (10):779–85.

20. Cobbe SM, Redmond MJ, Watson JM et al, 'Heartstart Scotland' – initial experience of a national scheme for out of hospital defibrillation, *Br Med J* (1991) **302** (6791):1517–20.

21. Michelucci A, Padeletti L, Frati M et al, Effects of ischemia and reperfusion on QT dispersion during coronary angioplasty, *PACE* (1996) **19** (Pt II):1905–8.

22. Sporton SC, Taggart P, Sutton PM et al, Acute ischaemia: a dynamic influence on QT dispersion, *Lancet* (1997) **349**:306–9.

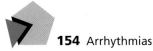

23. Campbell RWF, Murray A, Julian DG, The natural history of the first twelve hours of myocardial infarction, *Br Heart J* (1981) **46**:351–7.

24. Bourke JP, Young AA, Richards DAB et al, Reduction in incidence of inducible ventricular tachycardia after myocardial infarction by treatment with streptokinase during infarct evolution, *J Am Coll Cardiol* (1990) **16**:1703–10.

25. Volpi A, Cavalli A, Santoro E et al, Gruppo Italiano per lo Studio della Streptochinasi nell'Infarto Miocardico. Incidence and prognosis of secondary ventricular fibrillation in acute myocardial infarction. Evidence for a protective effect of thrombolytic therapy, *Circulation* (1990) **82**:1279–88.

26. Wilcox RG, Eastgate J, Harrison E et al, Ventricular arrhythmias during treatment with alteplase (recombinant tissue plasminogen activator) in suspected acute myocardial infarction, *Br Heart J* (1991) **65**:4–8.

27. Bigger JT, Fleiss JL, Kleiger R et al, The relationships among ventricular arrhythmias, left ventricular dysfunction, and mortality in the two years after myocardial infarction, *Circulation* (1984) **69**:250–8.

28. Farrell TG, Bashir Y, Cripps T et al, Risk stratification for arrhythmic events in postinfarction patients based on heart rate variability, ambulatory electrocardiographic variables and the signal-averaged electrocardiogram, *J Am Coll Cardiol* (1991) **18**:687–97.

29. May GS, Eberlein KA, Furberg CD et al, Secondary prevention after myocardial infarction: A review of long-term trials, *Prog Cardiovasc Dis* (1982) **24**:331–52.

30. Rehnqvist N, Olsson G, Erhardt L et al, Metoprolol in acute myocardial infarction reduces ventricular arrhythmias both in the early stage and after the acute event, *Int J Cardiol* (1987) **15**:301–8.

31. Pfisterer ME, Kiowski W, Brunner H et al, Long-term benefit of 1–year amiodarone treatment for persistent complex ventricular arrhythmias after myocardial infarction, *Circulation* (1993) **87** (2):309–11.

32. Marchlinski FE, Buxton AE, Waxman HL et al, Identifying patients at risk of sudden death after myocardial infarction: value of the response to programmed stimulation, degree of ventricular ectopic activity and severity of left ventricular dysfunction, *Am J Cardiol* (1983) **52**:1190–6.

33. Waller TJ, Kay HR, Spielman SR et al, Reduction in sudden death and total mortality by antiarrhythmic therapy evaluated by electrophysiologic drug testing: criteria of efficacy in patients with sustained ventricular tachyarrhythmia, *J Am Coll Cardiol* (1987) **10** (1):83–9.

34. O'Brien BJ, Buxton MJ, Rushby JA, Cost effectiveness of the implantable cardioverter defibrillator: a preliminary analysis, *Br Heart J* (1992) **68** (2): 241–5.

35. Sedgwick ML, Dalziel K, Watson J et al, The causative rhythm in out-of-hospital cardiac arrests witnessed by the emergency medical services in the Heartstart Scotland Project, *Resuscitation* (1994) **27** (1):55–9.

36. Wever EFD, Hauer RNW, van Capelle FJL et al, Randomized study of implantable defibrillator as first-choice therapy versus conventional strategy in postinfarct sudden death survivors, *Circulation* (1995) **91**:2195–203.

37. Cowan JC, Gardiner P, Reid DS et al, Amiodarone in the management of atrial fibrillation complicating myocardial infarction, *Br J Clin Pract* (1986) **40**:155–61.

38. Ormerod OJM, McGregor CJA, Stone DL et al, Arrhythmia after coronary bypass surgery, *Br Heart J* (1984) **51**:618–21.

39. Matangi MF, Nutze JM, Graham IS et al, Arrhythmia prophylaxis after aortocoronary bypass: the effect of mini dose propranolol, *J Thorac Cardiol Surg* (1985) **89**:439–43.

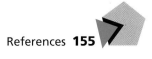

Chapter 6
The menopause

Michael Marsh

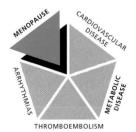

■ INTRODUCTION

The commonest cause of mortality in women living in industrialized societies is cardiovascular disease. Although mortality due to cardiovascular disease before 50 years of age is greater in men than in women, cardiovascular disease is an important cause of early death in women over 50. Over 50 per cent of post-menopausal women die from cardiovascular disease, and 80 per cent of these deaths are in women aged under 65 years. The incidence of myocardial infarction (MI) in women rises rapidly towards that of men after the menopause, and women have a 3–4-fold greater risk of atherosclerosis after a natural menopause. It is likely that the fall in endogenous oestrogens that occurs at the menopause is responsible for most of this increase in coronary heart disease (CHD).

The present chapter aims to address the following important questions:

• What is the evidence that hormone replacement therapy (HRT) (with or without progestogens) will reduce the risk of coronary disease in the general population of postmenopausal women?
• What is the evidence that HRT (with or without progestogens) will reduce the risk of MI in postmenopausal women with coronary artery disease (CAD)?
• What are the likely mechanisms for this effect?
• How do different types of HRT differ in their effect?

In the absence of satisfactory data from comparative studies of the effects of different types of HRT on the incidence of CAD, the last question can presently only be addressed by examining the effects of different types of HRT on risk markers for CAD. In women who have an intact uterus, HRT is usually administered in combination with progestogen to prevent endometrial carcinoma. Progestogens may oppose some of the effects of oestrogens on cardiovascular risk markers.

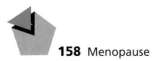

■ COMMONEST TYPES OF STEROIDS USED IN HRT

☐ Oestrogens

Oestrogens for systemic use may be administered orally, transdermally (by patch or cream) or as pellets of 17β-oestradiol for insertion under the skin. Conjugated equine oestrogens (CEE) form the most commonly used oral oestrogen preparation in HRT, and were the most commonly used type of oestrogen preparation in most long-term studies on the effects of oestrogens on CAD. This preparation incorporates a mixture of oestrogenic compounds, mainly oestrone sulphate and equilin sulphates. Oral micronized 17β-oestradiol is being increasingly used as an alternative to CEE. Oestradiol transdermal therapeutic systems (TTS) contain 17β-oestradiol dissolved in alcohol within a multilayered patch which is applied to the skin and changed twice a week. Recently, solid matrix patches incorporating 17β-oestradiol have become available. Different types of this patch can be changed once or twice a week. Crystalline implants containing 17β-oestradiol are inserted into the subcutaneous fat of the abdominal wall or buttock under local anesthetic every 3 or 6 months.

☐ Progestogens

In non-hysterectomized women, unopposed oestrogen therapy is associated with a 5–10-fold increase in risk of endometrial carcinoma. Progestogens prevent this effect and can be added to oestrogen to protect the endometrium either sequentially, i.e. for only a certain number of days per month (usually 12 or 14), or every day in a continuous combined regimen. Progestogens are most commonly given orally but some can be delivered transdermally. In future, progestogens will probably be available for transvaginal use or administration via an intrauterine device.

The clinically useful progestogens for HRT are (1) naturally occurring 21-carbon compounds, progesterone itself and its derivative 17-hydroxyprogesterone, (2) 21-carbon synthetic progesterone derivatives medroxyprogesterone acetate (MPA) and dydrogesterone, and (3) synthetic 19-nortestosterone derivatives norethisterone, norethisterone acetate and levonorgestrel

	Oestrogen	Progestogen
Sequential HRT		
With C19 progestogens		
Prempak C®	CEE	Norgestrel
Climagest®	Oestradiol valerate	Norethisterone
Nuvelle®	Oestradiol valerate	Levonorgestrel
Estrapak®	Transdermal oestradiol	Norethisterone
Estracombi®	Transdermal oestradiol	Transdermal norethisterone
Evoral Pak®	Transdermal oestradiol	Norethisterone
With C21 progestogens		
Premique® Cycle	CEE	MPA
Improvera®	PES	MPA
Femoston®	Oestradiol	Dydrogesterone
Femapak®	Transdermal oestradiol	Dydrogesterone
Continuous combined HRT		
With C19 progestogens		
Kliofem®	Oestradiol	Norethisterone
Climesse®	Oestradiol valerate	Norethisterone
With C21 progestogens		
Premique®	CEE	MPA

CEE = Conjugated equine oestrogens, PES = piperazone oestrone sulphate, MPA = medroxyprogesterone acetate.

Table 6.1 Examples of commercially available HRT preparations incorporating progestogens for non-hysterectomized women. Oral administration unless indicated.

and their 'third-generation' derivatives such as desogestrel, gestodene and norgestimate. A list of commercially available HRT combinations is given in Table 6.1.

■ OESTROGEN HRT

☐ What is the evidence that oestrogen replacement therapy (ERT) will reduce the risk of coronary disease in the general population of postmenopausal women?

Most case-controlled studies have shown a reduced risk of CAD in ERT users, although the results are not statistically significant in most (Figure 6.1). The relative risks from community based case-control studies range between 0.3 and 0.9.[1-3] The largest community-based study to date[1] studied 171 women (mean age 75 years), of whom 30 per cent were ever-users of ERT and 8.7 per cent current users. The relative adjusted risk of first MI for ever-users was 0.9 (CI 0.5–1.4) and for current users 0.7 (CI 0.3–1.4). In the follow-up study of 133 women[3] the relative risk of fatal MI using living controls was 0.4 (CI 0.2–0.8) and for dead controls was 0.6 (CI 0.3–1.0). Risk factor adjustment did not significantly alter these ratios.

Prospective studies have provided more substantial support for a cardioprotective effect of oestrogens. Bush and co workers[4] reported on the Lipids Research Clinics follow-up of 2270 women aged 40–69 years observed for an average of 8.5 years. The age-adjusted relative risk of MI among users compared with non-users was 0.34 (CI 0.12–0.81) and was largely unaffected by risk factor adjustment.

The Nurses Health Study[5] examined the effect of past versus present ERT use and CHD risk. In 1976, over 120 000 women aged 30–55 completed a questionnaire concerning health status, medical history, lifestyle, coronary risk factors and hormone use. The details were updated by questionnaires 2 and 4 years later. A total of 32 317 postmenopausal women with no history of CHD were followed for an average of 3.5 years. The relative risk of MI for ERT ever-users compared with never-users was 0.5 (CI 0.3–0.8). The

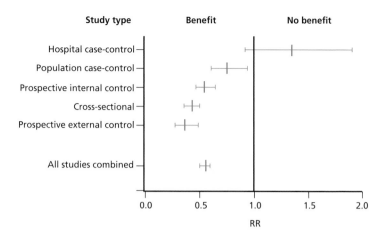

Figure 6.1 Relative risk and 95% confidence interval estimates of coronary disease associated with ERT use. (Modified with permission from Stampfer MJ, Colditz GA. Estrogen replacement therapy and coronary heart disease: a quantitative assessment of the epidemiological evidence. *Preventive Medicine* 1991; **20**; 47–63.)

relative risk in current users versus never-users was 0.3 (CI 0.2–0.6). The risk in past users versus never-users was 0.7, but was not significant, suggesting that the effects of oestrogen HRT on MI risk may decline after treatment is withdrawn. Adjustment for risk factors did not substantially change the risk estimates.

Further follow-up of these women for up to 10 years (337 854 person years) until 1986 gave similar results.[6] Current users had an adjusted relative risk of 0.56 (CI 0.4–0.8) for major coronary disease compared to never-users. The findings were similar in a low-risk group that excluded women reporting hypertension, current smoking, diabetes and hypercholesterolaemia, indicating that ERT may still produce beneficial effects in those at low risk of CAD.

Henderson et al[7] presented data from a study of 8841 women aged 40–101 years. After a mean 5.5 years of follow-up, 149 deaths due to MI occurred. The relative risk of fatal MI compared with never-users was 0.62 (CI 0.4–0.9) for past users, 0.5 (CI 0.2–1.1) for current users and 0.6 (CI 0.4–0.8) for ever-users. Risk factor adjustment had little effect on these figures.

Petitti et al[8] reported the results of 10–13 years follow-up of 6093 women aged 18–54 years. Cardiovascular disease mortality in ERT users was 0.9 (CI 0.2–3.3) compared with never-users.

In contrast to other studies, Wilson and colleagues[9] reported an increased risk of cardiovascular disease with ERT use in women taking part in the Framingham Heart Study. Oestrogen users were defined as women who were prescribed oestrogen at any time over an 8-year period. Follow-up for 8 years started at the end of this period for 1234 postmenopausal women aged 50 years or more, of whom 302 were classed as ERT users. The endpoints of cardiovascular disease were diverse, and included angina pectoris, intermittent claudication, transient ischaemic attack and congestive cardiac failure. After adjustment for age, obesity, alcohol consumption, smoking, hypertension, total cholesterol and high-density lipoprotein (HDL) cholesterol, the relative risk of cardiovascular disease for oestrogen users was 1.8 ($P < 0.01$). The initial report was criticized because oestrogen intake was not validated, for the failure to control for age and menopausal status in the analysis, and for the use of a wide range of endpoints. A reanalysis of the data[10] with an endpoint of CHD without angina showed a non-significant protective effect in women aged 50–59 years (relative risk 0.4) and a non-significant adverse effect in older women, in whom the relative risk was 2.2. In both Framingham reports the risk ratio was adjusted for HDL cholesterol levels, which is likely to be inappropriate, as HDL changes may be an important mechanism of oestrogen action.

Studies comparing the extent of coronary artery occlusion at arteriography between ERT users and non-users have shown less stenosis in ERT users. Sullivan et al[11] examined ERT usage in 1444 postmenopausal women with greater than 70 per cent coronary occlusion at angiography and in 744 women with no stenosis. Of the women with stenosis, 2.7 per cent used ERT, compared with 7.7 per cent of those without ($P < 0.01$). After adjustment for risk markers, the relative risk of stenosis for oestrogen users was 0.58 (CI 0.35–0.97). McFarland et al[12] using a similar study design in 283 postmenopausal women, found that the relative risk for severe versus no stenosis was 0.5 (CI 0.3–0.8).

☐ **What is the evidence that ERT will reduce the risk of myocardial infarction in postmenopausal women with coronary disease?**

There is some evidence that ERT will be beneficial to women who already have CAD. Sullivan and co-workers[13] retrospectively followed up for 10 years 2268 women aged over 55 years who had undergone angiography. The women were divided up into those with less than 70 per cent coronary artery stenosis ($n = 644$), those with more than 70 per cent stenosis ($n = 1178$) and those without stenosis ($n = 446$). The endpoint was mortality from all causes. At 10 years the survival for HRT users and never-users was 97 per cent and 60 per cent respectively ($P = 0.007$) in the group with the most severe stenosis. Significant differences between users and non-users were also seen in the women with less severe stenosis. However, the authors acknowledged that there were difficulties with the study. For example, never-users of HRT were older and smoked more than users.

More recently, the effect of ERT on survival after coronary artery bypass surgery has been reported.[14] The 10-year survival of untreated women was 65 per cent, whilst that of ERT users was 81.4% per cent.

■ OESTROGEN AND PROGESTOGEN HRT

□ What is the evidence that oestrogen and progestogen HRT will reduce the risk of coronary disease in the general population of postmenopausal women?

In most of the trials of the effects of HRT on MI risk, progestogen use was infrequent. However, in two prospective studies, progestogen use was more common. Hunt et al[15] examined mortality rates in 4544 postmenopausal women attending menopause clinics and compared them with those expected for the general female population of England and Wales, matched for age. Treated women had all taken HRT for at least 1 year, and 43 per cent of the treatments incorporated a progestogen. Recruitment started in 1978 and mortality from follow-up was assessed in 1984 and 1988. The relative risk of mortality from ischaemic heart disease was 0.48 at the first follow-up (CI 0.29–0.74) and 0.41 (CI 0.24–0.84) at the second.

Falkeborn et al[16] in a prospective cohort study, followed up 23 174 women for an average of 5.8 years. The median age at

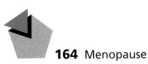

entry was 53.9 years. The endpoint was admission to hospital with first MI. The relative risk for HRT ever-users compared with never-users was 0.81 (CI 0.71–0.92). Of these women, 11 per cent had received progestogens. In women who were less than 60 years of age and received oral oestradiol/levonorgestrel HRT, the relative risk was 0.53 (CI 0.3–0.87).

Both of the above studies may be flawed by differences in risk factors for cardiovascular disease between women in the cohort and the comparison population. In the reports of Hunt et al, the study group was of higher social class than the general population. The HRT users in the study of Falkeborn et al practised more regular physical exercise, were leaner and were more highly educated.

There has been one clinical trial of oestrogen/progestogen HRT use on the CHD incidence.[17] Eighty-four pairs of women in a chronic care hospital, matched for age and medical condition, were randomized to take 2.5 mg conjugated oestrogen daily, to which was added 10 mg medroxyprogesterone acetate for 7 days a month, or to placebo. After 10 years of follow-up, the relative risk of fatal and non-fatal MI for treated women was 0.33 (CI 0.1–2.8). The result was statistically insignificant, possibly because of the low power of the study. There were only four MIs in the trial.

■ THE MECHANISMS FOR THE EFFECT OF HRT ON CHD

There are likely to be several mechanisms by which ERT reduces the risk of MI incidence. The effect of oestrogens on lipids and lipoproteins is undoubtedly important, but increasing evidence suggests that other actions of oestrogens are likely to be involved (Figure 6.2, Table 6.2).

☐ Effects of oestrogens on lipids and lipoproteins

Nearly all forms of oestrogen appear to increase HDL (especially HDL_2) and decrease LDL in postmenopausal women, depending

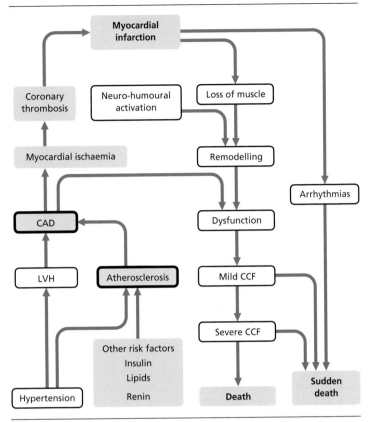

Figure 6.2 Impact of hormone replacement therapy on the ischaemic cycle.

on the dose, type and route of administration. Oestrogen treatment may also inhibit atheroma formation by reducing modifications to LDL, such as oxidation, that are thought to be important in atherogenesis.

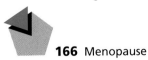

Decreases LDL cholesterol (oestrogens)
Increases HDL cholesterol (oestrogens)
Decreases triglyceride (progestogens)
Decreases LDL cholesterol oxidation (oestrogens)
Decreases LDL cholesterol uptake in blood vessels (oestrogens)
Decreases Lp(a) (oestrogens or progestogens)
Decreases vascular tone (oestrogens)
Preserves endothelial function (oestrogens)
Decreases formation of thromboxane A_2 (oestrogens)
Increases release of prostaglandin I_2 (oestrogens)
Improves insulin metabolism (oestrogens)
Improves body fat distribution (oestrogens)

Table 6.2 Possible mechanisms for cardioprotective effect of HRT.

☐ Oral oestrogens

A longitudinal study[18] of CEE 0.625 mg use reported a fall in total cholesterol of 4–8 per cent, a fall of 12–19 per cent of LDL and increases in HDL of 9–13 per cent following 3 months of treatment. Similar effects were seen in the cross-sectional study of Wahl et al[19] which compared 239 women taking a variety of regimens incorporating CEE with 370 controls matched for age, Body Mass Index (BMI), and cigarette and alcohol consumption. Women taking CEE had 13 per cent increase in HDL cholesterol levels, 25 per cent higher triglyceride levels and 14 per cent lower LDL cholesterol levels when compared to non-users.

The extent of the LDL-lowering effect of oestrogens used in HRT appears to be greatest in those women with the highest pretreatment levels. In the study of Tikkanen et al,[20] hyper- and normocholesterolaemic postmenopausal women were treated with 2 mg/day oestradiol valerate. HDL cholesterol levels rose and LDL levels fell, but LDL levels did not fall if pretreatment LDL was not raised.

There appears to be a dose-dependency effect of CEE on some lipoproteins. In a randomized, double-blind, crossover study,[21] treatment with CEE 0.625 mg/day produced a 15 per cent fall in LDL compared with placebo, but a higher dose of 1.25 mg/day produced only a slightly greater fall in LDL, of 19 per cent. HDL was 16 per cent and 18 per cent higher than placebo in the high- and low-dose groups respectively. The effect on total triglyceride appeared to be more clearly dose dependent. Triglyceride rose more in the higher-dose group, with an increase of 38 per cent compared with 24 per cent. This effect on triglyceride may be especially relevant in postmenopausal women, as serum triglyceride appears to be a risk marker for CHD in women.[22]

Two reports of the effects of CEE on lipoprotein (a) did not demonstrate an effect,[23,24] but Kim et al[25] studied 23 hysterectomized postmenopausal women who were given CEE 0.625 mg/day for 2 months and found that Lp(a) fell by approximately 26 per cent.

☐ Non-oral administration of oestrogens

Reports of the effects of subcutaneous 17β-oestradiol implants on plasma lipoproteins are conflicting. Lobo et al[26] demonstrated an increase of nearly 50 per cent in HDL using a 25-mg 17β-oestradiol pellet, but in a later study Stanczyk et al[27] did not detect such a large effect using two 25-mg implants, which only produced a rise of 10 per cent in HDL ($P < 0.05$). Farish et al[28] examined the effects of 50-mg pellets of 17β-oestradiol in 14 women over 6 months. A small fall in LDL cholesterol and increases in both HDL_2 and HDL_3 were seen.

Transdermal 17β-oestradiol probably causes changes in plasma lipoproteins that are different to those caused by oral therapy. Walsh et al[29] compared the effects of oral micronized oestradiol, 2 mg/day, and transdermal 17β-oestradiol, 100 μg/day. Oral therapy reduced LDL cholesterol by 14 per cent, increased HDL_2 by 39 per cent and increased total triglyceride by 24 per cent. The only effect of transdermal oestradiol was to increase HDL_2 by 23 per cent.

☐ Progestogens and lipids and lipoproteins

There have been many studies of the effects on plasma lipoproteins of oestrogen/progestogen HRT, but many studies are flawed by poor methodology or inadequate numbers. The results differ according to the oestrogen and progestogen dosage and type. In general, it appears that: (1) almost all progestogens will exert androgenic activity and cause a fall in HDL cholesterol if given in sufficiently high doses; (2) progestogens of higher androgenicity have the potentially beneficial effect of lowering triglycerides; and (3) the C21 progestogens have milder androgenic characteristics compared with C19 progestogens. The net result of oestrogens and progestogen combinations on lipoproteins therefore depends on the balance of the effects of these steroids.

☐ Formulations containing progesterone and C21 progestogens

Progesterone and progesterone derivatives appear to have little effect in opposing the plasma lipoprotein changes produced by the oestrogens used in HRT regimens.

van der Mooren et al[30] studied serum lipids and lipoproteins in 27 postmenopausal women after 6 and 12 months of treatment with 2 mg/day of micronized 17β-oestradiol, with dydrogesterone 10 mg/day added for 14 days each month. Six women had their dose of dydrogesterone increased to 20 mg to control vaginal bleeding during the trial. Serum was taken during the progestogen phase of treatment. At 6 months, compared with baseline, total cholesterol had fallen by 9 per cent and LDL by 16.3 per cent. HDL rose by 8 per cent and triglycerides by 14.4 per cent. These changes were maintained at 1 year.

In a multicentre study of similar design,[31] 235 postmenopausal women were treated with oral oestradiol 2 mg/day continuously and oral dydrogesterone 10 mg/day added for 14 out of every 28 days, and had lipid and lipoprotein levels measured at baseline and over 2 years. LDL fell by 15 per cent, HDL_2 rose by 33 per cent and triglyceride rose by 16 per cent.

Reports of the effects on lipids and lipoproteins of MPA when used in HRT are conflicting. One group[32] has reported that, when added to oestradiol valerate at 2 mg/day, MPA 10 mg/day for 10 days each cycle will lower HDL and HDL_2, whereas another group,[33] using the same formulation, reported no effect on HDL. There may have been differences in the bioavailability of the MPA between these studies.

MPA may have insufficient androgenic potency to reverse oestrogen effects if oestrogens are given in doses at the higher end of the therapeutic range. In a randomized double-blind study,[34] women were given either CEE 0.625 or 1.25 mg/day, combined with 10 days of either MPA 5 mg/day or placebo. In the groups given unopposed oestrogen, the higher oestrogen dose lowered LDL cholesterol (by 8 per cent), but both doses increased HDL cholesterol and triglycerides. With MPA addition, the progestogen prevented the increase in HDL seen with the low oestrogen dose formulation, which was then no different from baseline, but HDL remained raised with the higher oestrogen dose and was greater than baseline by 19 per cent at 1 year.

A recent 3-year prospective randomized double-blind placebo-controlled study[35] examined the effects of CEE 0.625 mg/day combined with MPA given either sequentially (10 mg/day for 12 days of every 28-day cycle) or continuously (2.5 mg day). Total triglyceride rose and LDL fell in all treatment groups. Although the changes in HDL in the MPA groups were less than in CEE users alone, all groups showed a rise in HDL compared with baseline, suggesting that MPA only weakly opposes HDL rises induced by oestrogen.

These findings are borne out by cross-sectional studies. In the report of Barret–Connor et al,[36] there were no differences in plasma lipoprotein levels between users of HRT oestrogen-only formulations and users of combined formulations containing MPA, although the number in the latter group (69) was small. Nabulsi et al[37] examined lipid and lipoprotein profiles of 5000 postmenopausal women, of whom approximately 20 per cent were taking HRT. Of the HRT users, about 20 per cent were using oestrogen and progestogen, mainly regimens of CEEs with sequential MPA. Users of HRT had significantly greater concentrations of HDL and triglyceride, and lower concentrations of LDL and Lp(a), than non-users. These differences were found for both oestrogen-only and oestrogen and progestogen therapies.

HRT regimens incorporating C21 progestogens probably cause a fall in Lp(a). Soma et al[38] reported a fall in Lp(a) in 10 women treated with CEE (1.25 mg/day) to which was added MPA 10 mg/day for 10 days of every 28-day cycle. van der Mooren et al[30] reported that cyclical 17β-oestradiol and dydrogesterone given over 1 year produced a 17.5 per cent fall in Lp(a). However, Muesing et al[23] did not find a significant effect on Lp(a) with CEE and MPA in 16 postmenopausal women. Kim et al[25] reported a much larger study of 132 postmenopausal women who received CEE 0.625 mg/day for 25 days out of 30, with MPA 5 mg/day added for 10 days in 65 women and MPA 10 mg/day in 67 women.

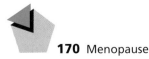

After 2 months of treatment, Lp(a) fell significantly by 14.7 per cent and 22.2 per cent in the high- and low-dose progestogen groups respectively.

☐ Formulations containing C19 progestogens and their derivatives

Oestradiol and norethisterone HRT combinations reduce LDL cholesterol, and high (e.g. 10 mg/day) or low (e.g. 1 mg/day) doses of norethisterone can counter the ability of oestrogens to increase HDL cholesterol, and have been reported to cause falls in HDL of approximately 20 per cent.[39,40]

The oestrogen dose appears to influence the effect of oestrogen/norethisterone combinations on plasma lipoproteins. Christiansen and colleagues[41] studied three groups of 10 postmenopausal women taking either 1, 2 or 4 mg/day micronized 17β-oestradiol, combined with 1 mg norethisterone for 10 days per cycle over two treatment cycles. HDL increased dose-dependently for samples taken during the oestrogen-only phase of treatment, with rises of approximately 4 per cent, 8 per cent and 16 per cent in increasing order of dosage. In the progestogen phase, HDL fell below baseline for the 1-mg group and rose approximately 4 per cent and 6 per cent above baseline for the 2- and 4-mg groups, respectively.

It appears that levonorgestrel, like norethisterone, opposes the increases in HDL produced by oestrogens and may cause a fall in HDL levels. A recent 3-year study[42] examined the effects of sequential regimens of oral (continuous CEEs, 0.625 mg/day. with *dl*-norgestrel 0.15 mg/day added for 12 days), or transdermal HRT (17β-oestradiol, 0.05 mg/day, with 0.25 mg/day norethisterone acetate added for 14 days). HDL was lower during the oestrogen/progestogen phase than during the oestrogen-only phase for both treatments. HDL fell in the reference group of women studied concurrently.

To summarize:
• oestrogens tend to increase HDL and lower LDL
• oral oestrogens increase triglycerides
• progestogens tend to counteract these effects to some extent depending on the type and dose of progestogen
• more androgenic C19 progestogens seem to counteract the beneficial oestrogenic effects to a greater extent

■ GLUCOSE METABOLISM

Insulin resistance and circulating insulin concentrations in women increase with age and years past the menopause, but are greater in postmenopausal women, independent of age.[43,44] Studies of 17β-oestradiol given to postmenopausal women suggest that pancreatic insulin secretion and insulin sensitivity is enhanced,[45,46] although alkylated oestrogens may raise insulin levels and impair glucose tolerance.[35,47]

A recent study has examined the effects on insulin resistance of oral and transdermal HRT regimens.[48] Healthy postmenopausal women were randomized to receive transdermal 17β-oestradiol 50 μg/day used in a sequential regimen with transdermal norethisterone acetate 250 μg/day or oral CEE 0.625 mg with sequential addition of dl-norgestrel 150 μg/day. An untreated reference group was studied concurrently. Both of these relatively androgenic progestogens caused an increase in insulin resistance. In contrast, a 2-year study of the effects of the relatively less androgenic C21 progestogen dydrogesterone used in a sequential regimen with oral 17β-oestradiol in 235 women demonstrated a fall in fasting insulin levels, no change in Oral Glucose Tolerance Test (OGTT) glucose responses and a fall in OGTT insulin responses, compatible with a reduction in insulin resistance.[31] This suggests that dydrogesterone does not oppose oestradiol-induced improvement in insulin sensitivity.

■ HAEMOSTASIS

It is unclear whether natural oestrogens have any clinically relevant effect on fibrinolytic/coagulation changes with oral HRT, but the most consistently demonstrated change has been a rise in factor VII_c. Some have reported rises in fibrinogen and factor X and a fall in antithrombin III levels.[49] One group has reported no change in serum fibrinogen levels over 3 years in women treated with a variety of oral HRT regimens, but a significant rise in fibrinogen in women treated with placebo.[35] Although data are sparse, non-oral HRT does not appear to influence fibrinolysis/coagulation.[50] At present, it seems likely that there is no clear favourable or unfavourable effect of ERT on thrombosis, although some recent reports suggest there may be a slight increase in risk.

■ OESTROGENS AND THE VASCULATURE

☐ Oestrogens and blood pressure

Oral natural oestrogens do not appear to cause a mean rise in blood pressure, although a small number (less than 2 per cent) of women will develop a significant rise at the beginning of therapy.[51] A recent 3-year prospective randomized double-blind placebo-controlled study examined the effect of HRT on blood pressure in 875 postmenopausal women.[35] Subjects were treated with CEE 0.625 mg/day combined with either MPA or micronized progesterone given sequentially or continuously. Over 3 years, mean systolic blood pressure rose in all groups, including those assigned to placebo. There were no significant differences in the mean change in systolic blood pressure between women receiving HRT and those receiving placebo. Mean diastolic blood pressure did not change. Other data suggest that blood pressure is lowered with HRT, but this is unlikely to be of sufficient magnitude to have an important effect on the development of CAD.

☐ Direct vascular effects of oestrogens and progestogens

Oestrogens are likely to have a direct effect on blood flow and arterial tone. Oestrogen receptor-associated protein has been found in the arterial wall muscularis,[52] and oestrogens are known to cause the release of vasoactive substances such as prostacyclin[53] and endothelium-derived relaxing factor.[54]

Oestradiol has an ionotropic effect in animals, increasing cardiac output and causing systemic vasodilatation.[55] Acute administration of oestrogen at a dose higher than those used in

HRT appears to have a beneficial effect on myocardial ischaemia in women with CAD.[56]

In a series of studies using Doppler ultrasound to measure parameters of flow, it has been demonstrated that oestrogens administered to postmenopausal women reduce the pulsatility index (PI), a measure of downstream impedance to flow, in the uterine[57,58] and internal carotid arteries.[59] The effect on the internal carotid artery occurs with oestrogens delivered either transdermally[59] or orally.[60] Reduced resistance to blood flow and increased vessel elasticity may reduce myocardial risk, either by reducing the likelihood of acute coronary artery vasospasm or by lessening atheroma formation.

It appears that progestogens can reverse the effects of oestrogens on vascular flow. In a study of sequential HRT incorporating norethisterone,[58] it was found that the uterine artery PI was higher (by approximately 13 per cent) during the oestrogen plus progestogen phase than during the oestrogen-only phase, but still remained lower (by approximately 33 per cent) than before treatment. A similar effect has also been reported in a study of carotid artery PI with the relatively less androgenic C21 progestogen, dydrogesterone.[61] It is possible that there are less marked differences between the C19 and C21 progestogens in effect on vascular tone than the clear differences seen with lipoproteins. Androgenicity may not be an important factor in the effect of different progestogens on vascular tone.

The time-course of the effect of norethisterone acetate on uterine artery PI has recently been reported.[62] Nine postmenopausal women were treated with either transdermal 17β-oestradiol 0.1 mg/day or CEE 1.25 mg/day, to which norethisterone acetate 0.7 mg/day was added for 12 days in a single 28-day cycle of therapy. The uterine artery PI was measured every 3–5 days over one treatment cycle. Compared with the oestrogen-only phase of the treatment cycle, norethisterone acetate increased the mean uterine artery PI by 30 per cent. Importantly, the PI fell significantly within 4 days of ceasing progestogen. Therefore, it appears that the progestogenic effect is short-lived. It is not known whether the time-course of the progestogenic effects observed in the uterine artery is seen throughout the systemic vasculature. If so, in regimens of continuous combined HRT, where oestrogen and progestogen are each given daily, progestogens may reduce the beneficial vascular effects of oestrogen on each day of treatment.

■ CLINICAL TRIALS OF HRT AND CARDIOVASCULAR DISEASE IN PROGRESS

A number of multicentre and single-centre trials of the effects of HRT on CHD mortality, morbidity and risk markers are presently underway. The Heart Estrogen/Progestin Replacement Study (HERS) is a randomized, double-blind, placebo-controlled study of premarin and MPA used in a continuous combined regimen. It is being conducted in 18 centres in the USA, and it is proposed that 2340 women will be followed for 5½ years. The endpoints include MI, stroke, need for coronary artery surgery and lipids and lipoproteins. The results are expected in the year 2000.

The Women's Health Initiative (WHI) study was set up by the National Institutes of Health (NIH) in the USA and aims to study the effects of dietary modification alone, calcium and vitamin D, CEE and MPA, CEE alone, or placebo, on CHD over 10 years. Women aged between 50 and 79 years are being recruited at 40 centres. It is planned that, in total, 164 000 women will be recruited, 64 000 of whom will be entered into the treatment arms and 100 000 into an observational study. The endpoints include CHD mortality and morbidity.

The European Trial of Estrogen/Progestin Replacement Treatment in the Post-menopause (EUTERP) is a multicentre double-blind placebo-controlled pilot study taking place in several European countries. Nine hundred women will be studied over 12 months and treated with continuous combined 17β-oestradiol and chlormadinone acetate or placebo. Four types of subjects will be recruited: women with type 1 or 2 diabetes, women with a history of deep vein thrombosis, women with a history of cardiovascular disease and women with no risk factors. Endpoints include serum lipids and lipoproteins and clotting factors. A follow-up larger multicentre European study of 4000 women is planned.

The Medical Research Council (MRC) trial is a randomized, double-blind study of the effects of HRT in 34 000 women, of whom 18 000 will be recruited in the UK. Treatment with HRT will last 10 years, with a further 10 years of follow-up. The endpoints include fatal and non-fatal MI, blood pressure and lipids and lipoproteins.

The Estrogen in the Prevention of Reinfarction Trial (ESPRIT) is a double-blind, multicentre, placebo-controlled study of the effect of oestradiol valerate on the risk of cardiac death or reinfarction in postmenopausal women. Women aged 50–69 years admitted with first MI to hospitals in the North West of England will be recruited. It is planned that a total of 2000 women will be studied for 30 months.

■ HRT – RISK AND BENEFITS

Full discussion of the risks and benefits of HRT, including the proven ability to reduce the risk of osteoporosis and its associated morbidity and mortality, is beyond the scope of this chapter. However, the risk of breast cancer with HRT is important and will be discussed, as both patients and prescribing physicians are especially concerned about this effect of HRT. The fear of developing breast cancer is a common reason for poor compliance.

Endogenous oestrogen exposure is known to affect risk of breast cancer. The lifetime risk is reduced in women who have undergone oophorectomy at an early age, and increased by early age at menarche, late menopause, nulliparity and obesity. It appears that the cumulative lifetime exposure to endogenous oestrogens is related to breast cancer risk.

The association between duration of exposure to oestrogens and breast cancer risk has also been reported with endogenous HRT use. Most studies comparing HRT non-users and women who have used HRT for 5 years or less have shown no increased risk of breast cancer. However, longer-term studies have reported an increased risk beyond 10 years of HRT use, with relative risks between 1.3 and 1.5. A dose-dependency effect has not been clearly seen.

The increased risk with duration of use probably does not raise the risk above that in the general population in women who have had a premature menopause and are using HRT until the natural age of menopause. In these women, the lifetime exposure to oestrogens is unlikely to be greater than that of women undergoing menopause at the usual age.

Importantly, most studies have not demonstrated increased mortality due to breast cancer with long-term HRT use. This is thought to be partly due to greater vigilance in the surveillance in HRT users compared with non-users, leading to earlier diagnosis and more successful treatment.

In summary, breast cancer risk, but not mortality, is probably increased with HRT when used for more than 10 years beyond the natural age at menopause. This information should be discussed with women when planning a strategy for long-term HRT use. It is important to ensure that women taking HRT are taught to correctly and regularly examine their own breasts, that they have yearly breast examinations by qualified staff and that they are strongly encouraged to take part in the national mammography screening programme.

■ CONCLUSIONS

There is substantial evidence that ERT will prevent CAD in the general population, and some data suggest that it will reduce cardiovascular mortality in women who already have CAD. However, the evidence concerning oestrogen/progestogen HRT use is scanty. The results of large randomized trials of the effects of oestrogen alone and oestrogen/progestogen HRT on myocardial disease risk are awaited. At present, risk matters for cardiovascular disease, such as lipids and lipoproteins, insulin resistance, body composition, haemostatic factors and vascular flow, have to be used as guidelines when prescribing oestrogen/progestogen HRT use to prevent cardiovascular disease in postmenopausal women. In non-hysterectomized women, it would seem sensible to use progestogens that have been shown to least adversely affect these risk markers at the lowest dosage needed to protect the endometrium and provide control of menstrual bleeding.

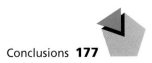

References

1. Pfeffer RI, Whipple GH, Kurosaki TT, Chapman JM, Coronary risk and oestrogen use in postmenopausal women, *Am J Epidemiol* (1978) **107**:479–87.

2. Bain C, Willett WC, Hennekens CH et al, Use of postmenopausal hormones and risk of myocardial infarction, *Circulation* (1981) **64**:42–6.

3. Ross RK, Paganini-Hill A, Mack TM et al, Menopausal oestrogen therapy and protection from ischaemic heart disease, *Lancet* (1981) **i**:858–60.

4. Bush TL, Barret-Connor E, Cowan LD et al, Cardiovascular mortality and noncontraceptive use of oestrogen in women: results from the Lipid Research Clinics Program Follow-up Study, *Circulation* (1987) **75**:1102–9.

5. Stampfer M, Willett W, Colditz G et al, A prospective study of postmenopausal estrogen therapy and coronary heart disease, *N Engl J Med* (1985) **313**:1044–9.

6. Stampfer MJ, Colditz GA, Estrogen replacement therapy and coronary heart disease: a quantitative assessment of the epidemiological evidence, *Prevent Med* (1991) **20**:47–63.

7. Henderson B, Paganini-Hill A, Ross R, Oestrogen replacement therapy and protection from acute myocardial infarction, *Am J Obstet Gynecol* (1988) **159**:27–31.

8. Petitti DB, Perlam JA, Sidney S. Non contraceptive oestrogens and mortality: long term follow-up of women in the Walnut Creek Study, *Obstet Gynecol* (1987) **70**: 289–93.

9. Wilson PWF, Garrison RJ, Castelli WP. Postmenopausal oestrogen use, cigarette smoking and cardiovascular mortality in women over 50: the Framingham study, *N Engl J Med* (1985) **313**:1038–43.

10. Eaker ED, Castelli WP, Coronary heart disease and its risk factors among women in the Framingham study, In: Eaker ED, Packard B, Wenger NK, Clarkson TB, Tyroler HA, eds, *Coronary Heart Disease in Women* (Haymarket Doyma Inc: New York, 1987).

11. Sullivan JM, Zwagg RV, Lemp GF et al, Postmenopausal oestrogen use and coronary atherosclerosis, *Ann Intern Med* (1988) **108**:358–63.

12. McFarland KF, Boniface ME, Hornung CA et al, Risk factors and non-contraceptive oestrogen use in women with and without coronary disease, *Am Heart J* (1989) **117**: 1209–14.

13. Sullivan JM, Zwagg RV, Lemp GF et al, Estrogen replacement and coronary artery disease: effect on survival in postmenopausal women, *Arch Intern Med* (1990) **150**: 2557–62.

14. Sullivan JM, El-Zeky F, Vander Zwaag R, Ramanathan KB, Oestrogen replacement therapy after coronary bypass surgery: effect on survival, *J Am Coll Cardiol* (1994) **23**:49A.

15. Hunt K, Vessy M, McPherson K, Mortality in a cohort of long-term users of hormone replacement therapy: an updated analysis, *Br J Obstet Gynecol* (1990) **97**:1080–6.

16. Falkeborn M, Persson I, Adami H-O et al, The risk of acute myocardial infarction after oestrogen and oestrogen–progestogen replacement, *Br J Obstet Gynaecol* (1992) **99**:821–8.

17. Nachtigall LE, Nachtigall RH, Nachtigall RD, Beckman EM, Oestrogen replacement therapy II: a prospective study in the relationship to carcinoma and cardiovascular and metabolic problems, *Obstet Gynecol* (1979) **54**: 74–9.

18. Miller VT, Muesing RA, LaRosa JC et al, Effects of conjugated equine oestrogens with and without three different progestogens on lipoproteins, high density lipoprotein subfractions and apolipoprotein A-I, *Obstet Gynecol* (1991) **71**: 235–40.

19. Wahl P, Walden C, Knopp R et al, Effects of oestrogen/progesterone potency on lipid/lipoprotein cholesterol, *N Engl J Med* (1983) **308**:862–7.

20. Tikkanen MJ, Kuusi T, Vartiainen E, Nikkila EA, Treatment of post-menopausal hypercholesterolaemia with oestradiol, *Acta Obstet Gynecol Scand (Suppl)* (1979) **88**:83–8.

21. Walsh BW, Schiff I, Rosner B et al, Effects of postmenopausal estrogen replacement on the concentrations and metabolism of plasma lipoproteins, *N Engl J Med* (1991) **325**:1196–204.

22. Lapidus L, Bengtsson C, Lindquist O et al, Triglycerides – main lipid risk factor for cardiovascular disease in women? *Acta Med Scand* (1985) **217**:481–9.

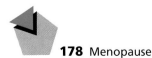

23. Muesing RA, Miller VA, Mills TM, LaRosa JC, Effects of postmenopausal unopposed estrogen and combined therapy on lipoprotein (a) levels, *Arterioscler Thromb* (1991) **11**:1452a.

24. Lobo RA, Notelovitz M, Bernstein L et al, Lp(a) lipoprotein – relationship to cardiovascular disease risk factors, exercise, and estrogen, *Am J Obstet Gynecol* (1992) **166**:1182–8.

25. Kim JK, Jang HC, Cho DH, Min YK, Effects of hormone replacement therapy on lipoprotein (a) and lipids in postmenopausal women, *Arterioscler Thromb* (1994) **14**:275–81.

26. Lobo R, March C, Goebelsmann U et al, Subdermal estradiol pellets following hysterectomy and oophorectomy, *Am J Obstet Gynecol* (1980) **138**:714–19.

27. Stanczyk FZ, Shoupe D, Nuunez V et al, A randomized comparison of nonoral estadiol delivery in postmenopausal women, *Am J Obstet Gynecol* (1988) **159**:1540–6.

28. Farish E, Fletcher C, Hart D et al, The effects of hormone implants on serum lipoproteins and steroid hormones in bilaterally oophorectomised women, *Acta Endocrinol* (1984) **106**:116–20.

29. Walsh BW, Schiff I, Rosner B et al, Effects of postmenopausal estrogen replacement on the concentrations and metabolism of plasma lipoproteins, *N Engl J Med* (1991) **325**:1196–204.

30. van der Mooren M, Demaker P, Thomas C, Rolland R, Beneficial effects on serum lipopoteins by 17β-oestradiol–dydrogesterone therapy in postmenopausal women: a prospective study, *Eur J Obstet Gynecol Reprod Biol* (1992) **47**:153–60.

31. Crook D, Multicentre evaluation of 17β oestradiol and dydrogesterone HRT on cardiovascular risk. In: *Abstracts of 8th International Congress on the Menopause* (1996) Sydney, F200, 106.

32. Ottoson UB, Johansson BG, von Schoultz B, Subfractions of high-density lipoprotein cholesterol during estrogen replacement therapy: a comparison between progestogens and natural progesterone, *Am J Obstet Gynecol* (1985) **151**:746–50.

33. Hirvonen E, Lipasti A, Malkonen M et al, Clinical and lipid metabolic effects of unopposed oestrogen and two oestrogen–progestagen regimens in postmenopausal women, *Maturitas* (1987) **9**:69–79.

34. Sherwin B, Gelfand MA, Prospective one-year study of estrogen and progestin in postmenopausal women: effects on clinical symptoms and lipoprotein lipids, *Obstet Gynecol* (1989) **73**: 759–66.

35. PEPI writing group, Effects of estrogen or estrogen/progestogen regimens on heart disease risk factors in postmenopausal women, *JAMA* (1995) **273**:199–208.

36. Barrett-Connor E, Wingard D, Criqui M, Postmenopausal estrogen use and heart disease risk factors in the 1980s. Rancho Bernardo, Calif, revisited, *JAMA* (1989) **261**:2095–100.

37. Nabulsi AA, Folsom AR, White A et al, Association of hormone replacement therapy with various cardiovascular risk factors in postmenopausal women, *N Engl J Med* (1993) **328**:1069–75.

38. Soma M, Fumagalli R, Paoletti R et al, Plasma Lp(a) concentration after oestrogen and progestagen in postmenopausal women, *Lancet* (1991) **337**:612.

39. Hirvonen E, Malkonen N, Manninen V, Effects of different progestogens on lipoproteins during postmenopausal replacement therapy, *N Engl J Med* (1981) **304**:562–5.

40. Mattsson LA, Cullberg G, Samsioe G, Evaluation of a continuous oestrogen–progestogen regimen for climacteric complaints, *Maturitas* (1982) **4**:95–102.

41. Jensen J, Nilas L, Christiansen C, Cyclic changes in serum cholesterol and lipoprotein following different doses of combined postmenopausal hormone replacement therapy, *Br J Obstet Gynaecol* (1986) **93**:613–18.

42. Whitcroft SI, Crook D, Marsh MS et al, Long-term effects of oral and transdermal hormone replacement therapies on serum lipid and lipoprotein concentrations, *Obstet Gynecol* (1994) **84**: 1–5.

43. Proudler AJ, Felton CV, Stevenson JC, Ageing and the response of plasma insulin, glucose and C-peptide concentrations to intravenous glucose in post-menopausal women, *Clin Sci* (1992) **83**:389–494.

44. Walton C, Godsland IF, Proudler A et al, The effects of the menopause on insulin sensitivity, secretion and metabolism in non-obese, healthy women, *Eur J Invest* (1993) **129**(suppl):466–73.

45. Notelovitz M, Johnston M, Smith S, Kitchens C, Metabolic and hormonal effects of 25 mg and 50 mg 17β estradiol implants in surgically menopausal women, *Obstet Gynecol* (1987) **70**: 749.

46. Cagnacci A, Soldani R, Carriero PL et al, Effects of low doses of transdermal 17β-oestradiol on carbohydrate metabolism in postmenopausal women, *J Clin Endocrinol Metab* (1992) **74**:1396–400.

47. Spellacy W, Buhi W, Birk S, The effects of estrogens on carbohydrate metabolism: glucose, insulin and growth hormone studies on one hundred and seventy one women ingesting Premarin, mestranol and ethinyl estradiol for six months, *Am J Obstet Gynecol* (1972) **114**:378–92.

48. Godsland I, Gangar KF, Walton C et al, Insulin resistance, secretion and elimination in postmenopausal women receiving oral or transdermal hormone replacement therapy, *Metabolism* (1993) **42**:846–53.

49. Stanwell-Smith R, Meade TW, Hormone replacement therapy for menopausal women: a review of its effects on haemostatic function, lipids and blood pressure, *Adv Drug React Acute Poisoning Rev* (1984) **4**:187–210.

50. Fox J, John George J, Newton J et al, The effect of transdermal oestradiol on haemostatic balance of menopausal women, *Maturitas* (1993) **18**:55–64.

51. Wren BG, Brown LB, Routledge DA, Differential clinical response to oestrogens after the menopause, *Med J Aust* (1982) **2**:329.

52. Padwick M, Whitehead M, Coffer A, King R, Demonstration of oestrogen receptor related protein in female tissues. In: Studd JWW, Whitehead MI, eds. *The Menopause* (Blackwell Scientific: Oxford, 1988) 227–233.

53. Steinleitner A, Stanczyk F, Levin J et al, Decreased in-vitro production of six-keto-prostaglandin F1 alpha on uterine arteries of postmenopausal women, *Am J Obstet Gynecol* (1989) **161**:1677–81.

54. Gisclard V, Millar V, van Houte P, Effects of 17 beta oestradiol on endothelium-dependent responses in the rabbit, *Pharmacol Exp Ther* (1988) **244**:19–22.

55. Magness RR, Rosenfeld CR, Local and systemic estradiol-17 beta: effects on uterine and systemic vasodilation, *Am J Physiol* (1989) **256**:E536–42.

56. Rosano GMC, Sarrel PM, Poole-Wilson PA, Collins P, Beneficial effects of oestrogen on exercise-induced myocardial ischaemia in women with coronary artery disease, *Lancet* (1993) **342**:133–6.

57. Bourne T, Hillard T, Whitehead M et al, Evidence for a rapid effect of oestrogens on the arterial status of postmenopausal women, *Lancet* (1990) **335**:1470–1.

58. Hillard TC, Bourne TH, Whitehead MI et al, Differential effects of transdermal estradiol and sequential progestogens on impedance to flow within the uterine arteries of postmenopausal women, *Fertil Steril* (1992) **58**:959–63.

59. Gangar KF, Vyas S, Whitehead MI et al, Pulsatility index in the internal carotid artery is influenced by transdermal estradiol and time since menopause, *Lancet* (1991) **338**:839–42.

60. Marsh MS, Ross D, Whitcroft SIJ, Ellerington M, Witehead MI, Oral oestradiol HRT reduces internal carotid artery pulsatility index in postmenopausal women, In: *Abstracts of the British Menopause Society Conference* (1994), York.

61. Cooper A, Ross D, Spencer C, Marsh MS, Stevenson JC, Whitehead MI, An open study of the effects of oral 17-β oestradiol and oral dydrogesterone on the internal carotid artery pulsatility index in hysterec-tomised women. In: *Abstracts of 8th International Congress on the Menopause* (1996) Sydney, P140, 160.

62. Marsh MS, Bourne TH, Whitehead MI et al, The temporal effect of progestogen on the uterine artery pulsatility index in postmenopausal women receiving sequential hormone replacement therapy, *Fertil Steril* (1994) **62**:771–4.

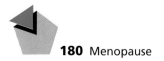

Chapter 7
Cardioprotection – the future

Richard Horton

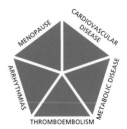

The tendency for medicine to progress in terms of the latest fashion is especially noticeable in cardiology. As the technical means for observing (angioscopy), physically removing (laser angioplasty) and revascularizing (stents) coronary atheroma have developed at a remarkable pace, so the notion that judicious pharmacological intervention alone can preserve myocardium and save lives has receded into relative obscurity.

We have tried to show the clinical importance of intervention in five simple but pre-eminent areas that can bring about substantial reductions in cardiovascular morbidity and mortality. We believe that there is a need for a new way of managing patients with or at risk of coronary artery disease (CAD). To this end, we have suggested the phrase 'cardioprotective therapeutics' to underline this new concept.

Cardioprotective therapeutics straddles various specialities: cardiology, diabetes, angiology, lipidology, clinical pharmacology and gynaecology. None of these taken alone adequately covers the single broad category of cardioprotection. If the long-term management of patients with (subclinical) CAD is to succeed in preventing further episodes of major cardiac decline, this integrated approach is essential. We believe that our pentagon of protection draws attention – hopefully in a memorable way – to the management of the complex influences operating in the course of ischaemic heart disease.

But one question may still trouble the sceptical reader: what is cardioprotection?

Kubler and Haas have presented the most detailed and rigorous analysis of the cardioprotective concept.[1] They define cardioprotection as, 'all mechanisms and means that contribute to the preservation of the heart by reducing or even preventing myocardial damage'. This broad view encompasses various medical and surgical interventions, across both primary and secondary prevention. First, there are *adaptive and compensatory physiological mechanisms* that contribute to the preservation of heart tissue. These mechanisms are summarized in Table 7.1; the principles that follow from them are important to keep in the back of one's mind but they are not directly clinically relevant.

Second, *therapeutic interventions* that promote cardioprotection include attention to all five aspects of management – vascular (hypertension and ischaemic heart disease); metabolic (lipids and diabetes); thromboembolic; arrhythmias; and the menopause. In particular, they represent, in the acute setting, thrombolysis,

Acute mechanisms

Regulation of oxygen supply:
  Myocardial work can only be increased if blood flow changes immediately on demand. Normally, this adaptation takes place at a coronary venous PO_2 of 20 mmHg; the PO_2 at which myocardial metabolism becomes threatened is 5 mmHg. Adaptation occurs well above the critical levels of PO_2

Adaptation of metabolic flow rates:
  To ensure instant shifts in energy supply to match demand, regulatory enzymes are activated simultaneously under ischaemic stress. Immediate generation of lactate and ATP is the result

High reserve capacity of key functions:
  The metabolic reserve of the heart can exceed demand by as much as 100 per cent, even under maximum stimulation

Multistage control of protective pathways:
  Several mechanisms exist – e.g. activation of presynaptic α_2–receptors – to damp down sympathetic activity

Ischaemic preconditioning:
  Short intervals of cardiac ischaemia can produce myocardial tolerance to subsequent episodes of stress

Chronic mechanisms

Neurohormonal activation:
  In early left ventricular impairment, sympathetic activation can improve function. Benefit may turn to damage as left ventricular function worsens

Left ventricular hypertrophy and dilatation:
  Both of these factors substantially increase the risk of mortality

Hibernating myocardium:
  Hibernation is a reversible impairment of myocardial function at rest which diminishes metabolic demand

Table 7.1 Physiological adaptive and compensatory mechanisms contributing to cardioprotection.

PTCA, emergency aortic valve replacement, and the use of cardioplegia during cardiac surgery. Patients with congestive heart failure and coronary disease will also benefit from more chronic management. It is in this longer-term scenario that a cardioprotective focus in treatment decisions may give particular rewards. What are the recent trends in these two aspects of clinical care?

■ CARDIOPROTECTION AND HEART FAILURE

☐ Carvedilol

The results of both V-HeFT I (hydralazine and isosorbide dinitrate) and V-HeFT II (ACE inhibitor) – the Veterans Heart Failure Trials[2,3] – showed the benefit of both peripheral vasodilatation and afterload reduction on outcome in patients with heart failure.

One especially promising recent advance has come with carvedilol, a beta-blocker with alpha₁–blocking vasodilator properties, together with antioxidant and other anti-ischaemic effects. The largest single placebo-controlled trial to investigate the efficacy of this agent in patients with congestive heart failure secondary to ischaemic heart disease was reported in 1997.[4] This study is summarized in Figure 7.1. After 12 months, left ventricular ejection fraction had increased by 5.3 per cent (2p < 0.0001) in the carvedilol group. Although after 19 months the frequency of worsening heart failure was similar in the placebo and carvedilol groups, the rate of death or hospital admission was reduced in those receiving carvedilol (104 versus 131; RR 0.74(0.57–0.95)).

Carvedilol has no demonstrable effect on exercise performance, symptoms, or episodes of worsening cardiac failure. However, there was an overall reduction of cardiovascular and clinical events with this drug. This single study confirmed the combined data of four small US trials.[5] The authors of the *Lancet* paper concluded that, when results from larger mortality trials became available, 'carvedilol has the potential to become part of standard therapy for many patients with heart failure'.

Patients registered 447

Patients eligble 442

Randomized 415

Carvedilol 207			Placebo 208		
Cause of death					**Relative risk (95%CI)**
Heart failure	14		15		0.92 (0.45–1.91)
MI	4		5		0.79 (0.21–2.94)
All deaths	18		20		0.89 (0.47–1.68)
Non-CV death	2		6		0.32 (0.07–1.60)
All deaths	20		26		0.76 (0.42–1.36)
Cause of hospital admission					
Heart failure	23		33		0.68 (0.40–1.17)
Ischaemic heart disease	25		34		0.70 (0.42–1.18)
Other CV disease	40		38		1.07 (0.68–1.66)
All CV disease	70		83		0.82 (0.59–1.12)
Non-CV disease	51		69		0.70 (0.49–1.01)
All admissions	99		120		0.77 (0.59–1.00)

Figure 7.1 The Australian/New Zealand Carvedilol Trial.[4]

☐ Ibopamine

Enthusiasm for new drugs that may influence peripheral cardio-vascular and direct cardiac function (as for carvedilol) needs to be tempered by a realistic appraisal of data from well-powered trials. One such trial is PRIME II – the second prospective randomized study of ibopamine on mortality and efficacy.[6] Ibopamine is a dopamine receptor (DA-1 and DA-2) agonist; it also causes renal and peripheral vasodilatation. Small clinical studies had suggested that this drug improved both symptoms and exercise tolerance in patients with mild-to-moderate heart

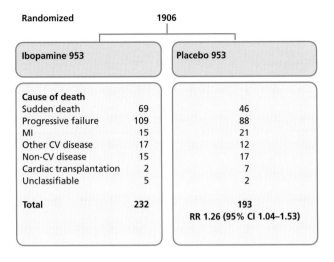

Figure 7.2 Ibopamine in patients with advanced severe heart failure.[6]

failure. The study design and summary outcome measures of PRIME II are shown in Figure 7.2. The trial was stopped early on the advice of the study safety committee. There was a significant increase in the number of deaths among patients taking ibopamine. The precise reasons remain unclear.

In an accompanying editorial to the full publication of PRIME II, Niebauer and Coats argued a strong line favouring caution:[7]

In view of the number of promising drugs that have eventually been shown to have a detrimental effect on survival in severe CHF, it may be time for a moratorium on human studies that investigate stimulatory drugs of the catecholamine receptor and their post-receptor pathways until convincing animal data show chronic survival benefit.

☐ Amiodarone

For other drugs, the results of clinical trials may not be clear-cut one way or the other. This is true for amiodarone in the treatment of patients with congestive heart failure. Two small trials – GESICA[8] and CHF-STAT[9] – had indicated substantial risk reductions in sudden death, progression of heart failure, left ventricular ejection function, and hospital admissions for patients receiving amiodarone. CHF-STAT was less promising and did not support the routine use of amiodarone in patients with heart failure. Nevertheless, great hope was placed in two large randomized trials – EMIAT[10] and CAMIAT.[11] Amiodarone reduced risk of arrhythmic death in both trials. However, neither study revealed any differences in all-cause mortality. Two forthcoming meta-analyses may throw further – perhaps more positive – light on the question of overall survival benefit.

☐ Losartan

The efficacy of angiotensin-converting enzyme (ACE) inhibitors has mostly been attributed to reduced angiotensin II production. Direct angiotensin II antagonists might therefore be thought to exhibit beneficial effects in patients with heart failure. Furthermore, since they do not reduce the breakdown of bradykinin, which might be responsible for some of the adverse effects of ACE inhibitors, angiotensin II antagonists might have advantages.

The primary endpoint of ELITE[12] – the Evaluation of Losartan in the Elderly Study – was a measure of tolerability of serum creatinine to the drug. A secondary endpoint was a composite efficacy measure of death and/or hospital admission. A summary of the trial design and outcomes is shown in Figure 7.3. Persisting changes in serum creatinine occurred in both groups equally after 48 weeks of follow-up. Fewer adverse events were reported in the losartan group (12.2 per cent versus 20.8 per cent; $p = 0.002$). Remarkably, in this small trial there was a large and significant difference in all-cause mortality among those receiving losartan. A larger trial to assess this effect as a primary outcome measure is in progress.

☐ Digoxin

Digitalis has been prescribed for patients with heart failure for over 200 years. Yet its cardioprotective effects have remained

Randomized		722		

Losartan 352			Captopril 370	

Combined death and/or admission for heart failure	33		Risk reduction (95%CI) 49 0.32 (−0.04–0.55)

	Losartan		Captopril	Risk reduction (95%CI)
Combined death and/or admission for				
heart failure	33		49	0.32 (−0.04–0.55)
All deaths				
Cardiovascular	17		32	0.46 (0.05–0.69)*
Sudden death	5		14	0.64 (0.03–0.86)
Progressive failure	1		1	−0.11 (−20.23–0.94)
MI	1		4	0.76 (−0.83–0.97)
Other	5		5	−0.03 (−2.63–0.71)
Non-cardiovascular	5		8	0.35 (−0.94–0.78)
Hospital admission				
Heart failure	20		21	0.04 (−0.74–0.47)
Any reason	78		110	0.26 (0.05–0.43)+

* $p = 0.035$
\+ $p = 0.014$

Figure 7.3 Evaluation of Losartan in the Elderly Study (ELITE).[12]

obscure until only very recently. The landmark DIG (Digitalis Investigation Group) trial[13] randomized over 6000 patients with heart failure (over two-thirds NYHA class I and II) to either digoxin or placebo, in addition to diuretics and ACE inhibitors (Figure 7.4). Digoxin failed to produce reductions in overall mortality, although the rates of both worsening heart failure and hospitalizations did decline.

These results are not entirely helpful for the clinician. Although survival is unaffected, there may be sufficient symptomatic benefit to justify use of digoxin. Moreover, the majority of the patient population, although they all had left ventricular ejection fractions of 0.45 or less, did not have severe heart failure according to the NYHA classification. For this

Digoxin 3397

Placebo 3403

Deaths	Digoxin	Placebo	Risk ratio (95%CI)
Total	1181	1194	0.99 (0.91–1.07)
Cardiovascular	1016	1004	1.01 (0.93–1.10)
Worsening CHF	394	449	0.88 (0.77–1.01)
Other cardiac	508	444	1.14 (1.01–1.30)
Other vascular	50	45	1.11 (0.74–1.66)
Hospitalizations			
Total	2184	2282	0.92 (0.87–0.98)*
Cardiovascular	1694	1850	0.87 (0.81–0.93)+
Worsening CHF	910	1180	0.72 (0.66–0.79)+
Digoxin toxicity	67	31	2.17 (1.42–3.32)+
Cardiac arrest	142	145	0.98 (0.78–1.24)
MI	195	201	0.97 (0.79–1.18)
Stroke	157	1164	0.95 (0.77–1.19)

* $p = 0.006$
+ $p < 0.001$

Figure 7.4 The Digitalis Investigation Group Trial.[13]

group, the physician must still practise with the eye of faith, at least regarding the use of digoxin. Further evidence for this group is needed. The last word on the cardioprotective effects of digoxin may reasonably be left to Milton Packer:[14]

'What will change as a result of the publication of this trial? For most patients with heart failure, digitalis remains an effective, safe, and inexpensive choice for the relief of symptoms, despite its inability to alter the natural history of the disease. To the extent that symptom relief has driven most of the drug's clinical use, the results of the trial should not lead most physicians to change their prescribing patterns. Nor will the results of the trial resolve the 200–year-old controversy surrounding the drug.'

■ CARDIOPROTECTION AND CORONARY ARTERY DISEASE

Kubler and Haass identify three key endpoints when evaluating cardioprotective efficacy in patients with coronary disease: first, symptomatic improvement; second, diminution of myocardial ischaemia; and third, reduction in mortality.

☐ Drugs

The main classes of drug that are used to treat coronary disease either symptomatically or directly are:

- nitrates
- calcium channel blockers
- beta-blockers
- statins

A detailed discussion of these drug classes can be found in earlier chapters. I would like to comment briefly on one aspect of this complex and controversial domain. The position of calcium antagonists remains uncertain, mainly because there is a small amount of randomized evidence proving their safety or danger one way or another. At the time of writing only four randomized trials exist to throw light on the question of calcium antagonist safety – namely, MIDAS,[15] PRAISE,[16] DEFIANT II[17] and CRIS[18] (Table 7.2). Much has been made of observational epidemiological evidence; this work is inevitably inconclusive and can be safely set aside from the present discussion. The clinical trial that raised the greatest anxiety was MIDAS – the Multicentre Isradipine Diuretic Atherosclerosis Study.

This randomized, double-blind study set out to investigate the rate of progression of intimal–media thickness in 12 carotid focal points over a 3-year period. Patients were randomized to receive either the short-acting calcium antagonist isradipine ($n = 442$) or hydrochlorothiazide ($n = 441$). There was no difference between the two groups in the rate of progression of mean maximum intimal–media thickness. However, there was an unexpected higher frequency of major vascular events (eg, MI, sudden death, stroke) among those taking isradipine ($n = 25$, 5.65 per cent) compared with those taking the diuretic ($n = 14$,

Trial	Intervention	Patients included	n	Primary outcome measure	Interpretation
MIDAS[15]	Isradipine versus hydrochlorothiazide	Diastolic hypertension	883	Rate of progression of mean maximum IMT in 12 carotid focal points at 3 years	Increased incidence of major and non-major vascular events
PRAISE[16]	Amlodipine versus placebo	Severe chronic heart failure	1153	Death from any cause and hospital admission for major vascular events	Amlodipine is safe; possible prolonged survival in those with non-ischaemic dilated cardiomyopathy
DEFIANT II[17]	Nisoldipine versus placebo	Post-acute MI	542	Aspects of exercise activity	Safe; no improvement in exercise time
CRIS[18]	Verapamil versus placebo	Acute MI	1775	All-cause mortality	No effect of verapamil was found

IMT = intimal–media thickness; MI = myocardial infarction.

Table 7.2 Randomized evidence and the safety of calcium channel blockers.

3.17 per cent), although this difference was non-significant (p = 0.07). There was also a significant increase in non-major vascular events and procedures (e.g. transient ischaemic attack, aortic-valve replacement) in the isradipine group (40 (9.05 per cent) versus 23 (5.22 per cent); p = 0.02).

PRAISE (with amlodipine), DEFIANT II (nisoldipine), and CRIS (verapamil) all failed to find any adverse effect. In addition, the Shanghai trial of nifedipine in the elderly (STONE), though non-randomized, also failed to identify any adverse risk.[19] The final answer about safety will come from large randomized trials, notably Syst-Eur and HOT (the Hypertension Optimal Treatment Study[20]). The final results of the Syst-Eur (Systolic Hypertension in Europe) trial revealed that treatment with nitrendipine (enalapril and hydrochlorothiazide added as necessary) reduced stroke incidence by 42% (p=0.003). Importantly, all combined fatal and non-fatal cardiovascular endpoints were reduced by a third and this decrease was also statistically significant (see Figure 7.5).[21]

The peculiar recent focus on calcium antagonist safety reflects the huge and largely unqualified enthusiasm with which clinicians prescribed these drugs in preceding years. By contrast, beta-blockers have become relatively unfashionable. Yet Kennedy and Rosenson[22] have discussed this issue with reference to prescribing patterns in the USA. An overestimation of the adverse effects of beta-blockers and an underappreciation of their efficacy were the main reasons for the persistent bias against their use, they conclude. However, Kennedy and Rosenson also point out that

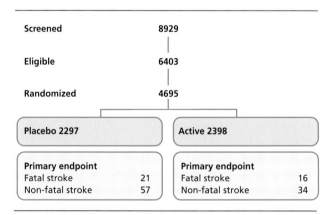

Figure 7.5 The Syst-Eur study.[21]

practice is changing. During the past 10 years or so, the frequency of beta-blocker use has more than doubled. It is worth pondering, at some length, on their interpretation of these events:

'... it must be realised that commercial influence in the lucrative pharmaceutical competitive marketplace of the North American continent has also contributed to negative attitudes of physicians regarding beta-blocker therapy ... . It is our experience that frequently in the past, all beta-blockers were 'lumped' by pharmaceutical competitors into a pharmacologic category associated with 'harmful lipid effects', 'decreased sexual function', 'increased heart failure' or 'decreased exercise performance'. In reality, such claims were often exaggerated, unsubstantiated or untrue and rarely applied to the majority of beta-blocking agents. Nevertheless, it appears that many physicians were susceptible to such medical concerns and chose another class of pharmaceutical agents to avoid potential therapeutic complications. We speculate that this 'switch class' tactic has in part contributed to the documented frequent use of calcium channel blocking agents and relative non use of beta-blockers in patients with ischaemic heart disease in North America.'

The platelet and coagulation systems are also therapeutic targets that will continue to generate interest for their cardioprotective potential. Thrombin inhibitors and IIb/IIIa receptor blockers show particular promise.[23] For example, the CAPTURE study (c7E3 Fab Anti-Platelet Therapy in Unstable Refractory Angina) found that the platelet IIb/IIIa antagonist c7E3 (abciximab) reduced the incidence of MI and urgent reintervention among 1265 patients with unstable angina undergoing PTCA.[24]

One should pause for thought here also. As with heart failure, not all trials in patients with coronary disease have such a clearly positive outcome. CAPRIE (clopidogrel versus aspirin in patients at risk of ischaemic events) is a good example.[25] This study was designed to assess the long-term efficacy of a ticlopidine-like agent, clopidogrel, among patients with atherosclerotic vascular disease (ischaemic stroke, MI and peripheral arterial disease). Over 19 000 patients were recruited, with a mean follow-up of 1.91 years. The risk of one of the clinical endpoints occurring was 5.32 per cent in the group treated with clopidogrel versus 5.83 per cent among those treated with aspirin (p= 0.043). Though statistically significant, the clinical value of this difference is negligible – and frankly disappointing. The authors made a great deal of the differences between the three vascular disease groups, but no cardioprotective benefit was truly apparent.

☐ Interventions

The main clinical questions regarding intervention focus on how to prevent restenosis following successful revascularization of an occluded coronary artery. Cardiac stents offer an especially enticing avenue.[26] First conceived by Alexis Carrel, who implanted glass and metal tubes into the aortas of dogs, the modern coronary stent is approaching routine use. Long-term data on restenosis rates are still being gathered, and thrombosis and neo-intimal hyperplasia remain important complications, but early results look promising.

An example is BENESTENT II. This randomized trial tested a heparin-coated stent in patients with multilesion, multivessel disease. In the trial, 827 patients were randomized to undergo either angioplasty ($n = 413$) or stent placement ($n = 414$). When rates of major adverse cardiac events – death, acute MI, bypass surgery, and reangioplasty – were measured at 15 days, there was no significant difference between stent placement and angioplasty (4.3 per cent versus 6.5 per cent). The presence of heparin and the use of a ticlopidine/aspirin regimen after stenting produced a subacute coronary occlusion rate of only 0.2 per cent (one patient) compared with a 1.7 per cent occlusion rate in those undergoing angioplasty. Bleeding complications were no different between the two groups.

In the routine setting, bail-out stenting has strikingly reduced the need for emergency coronary bypass following balloon angioplasty. Enthusiastic interventionists are also tending to place stents where balloon angioplasty is suboptimal (conditional stenting). This wave of fashionable optimism stems mainly from two important clinical trials – namely, STRESS[27] and BENESTENT I.[28] Also, among patients who experienced complications following angioplasty for acute MI, stent implantation seems a valuable way of restoring vessel patency[29].

Restenosis may also prove amenable to manipulation with platelet IIb/IIIa antagonists. For instance, in the IMPACT II study,[30] 4010 patients undergoing elective, urgent, emergency coronary intervention were randomized to receive one of three treatments: placebo, integrilin (135 μg/kg plus 0.5 μg/kg/min

	Aggressive strategy	Conservative strategy
Mortality at hospital discharge (mean 9 days)	21	6
Mortality at 1 month	23	9

Table 7.3 VANQWISH: final results, a cause for concern.

infusion for 20–24 h) or integrilin (135 μg/kg plus 0.75 μg/kg/min infusion). Integrilin (135/0.5 regimen) provided a 19 per cent non-significant reduction in the primary composite endpoint of 30-day death, MI or revascularization. When these data were analysed by actual treatment received (a planned secondary endpoint), the difference between integrilin and placebo reached significance (p = 0.035). These results are encouraging but hardly striking. Nevertheless, the platelet IIb/IIIa receptor is likely to be a continued source of intense investigation.

The generally positive tone that surrounds reports of increasingly aggressive interventional strategies was somewhat punctured by the results of the VANQWISH (VA Non-Q Wave in Hospital) trial. These data were reported at the 1997 annual meeting of the American College of Cardiology.[31] VANQWISH enrolled 920 patients with a diagnosis of non-Q-wave MI. On discharge from the coronary care unit, patients were randomized to undergo either an aggressive or a conservative follow-up strategy. Patients in the 'aggressive' group had an angiogram immediately, whilst those in the 'conservative' arm had a comprehensive programme of non-invasive testing (thallium stress test and radionuclide ventriculogram). Only if non-invasive testing revealed evidence of ischaemia was an angiogram performed; otherwise patients were treated medically. The results, shown in Table 7.3, speak for themselves.

■ INSIGHTS FROM BASIC SCIENCE

More fundamental laboratory approaches that are likely to reveal therapeutic benefits are almost impossible to predict. For example, in the first edition of this book (1994), we wrote about the then eye-catching prospects of the ACE gene. That story fell flat on its face in subsequent years. However, I will attempt a little crystal-ball gazing; if nothing else, this will serve as a useful benchmark for critics (and myself) in later years.

☐ Insulin resistance

The results of the Insulin Resistance and Atherosclerosis Study[32] showed a tight relation between vascular intimal–media thickness and differences in insulin sensitivity. As Reaven and Chen noted.[33] 'The sooner insulin resistance and its consequences become accepted as "traditional" risk factors for CHD, the better.' The treatment opportunities likely to ensue remain elusive at present.

☐ Homocysteine

Homocysteine is a metabolite of methionine. In patients with hyperhomocysteinaemia, there are atherogenesis and prothrombotic tendencies. Homocysteine has a toxic effect on endothelium, and platelet survival may be impaired. Evidence suggests that homocysteine may be an independent risk factor for vascular disease.[34] Folic acid reduces plasma homocysteine concentrations. It may yet be proven to offer therapeutic benefit.

☐ Ischaemic preconditioning

Preconditioning is a physiological process in which short intervals of sublethal ischaemia reduce subsequent damage to the heart during prolonged coronary occlusion.[35] The goal is to discover 'preconditioning mimetics'.

☐ Nitric oxide

NO is an important contributor to cardiovascular homeostasis. However, in certain circumstances, its modulation through inhibition of one or more forms of NO synthase may offer therapeutic advantages. For example, if inducible NOS is involved in inflammatory damage to the vessel wall, its specific inhibition may provide a means to retard the coronary lesion. Bhagat and Vallance have reviewed this possibility[36] and seem cautiously optimistic.

☐ Autonomic nervous system

In many respects, sudden cardiac death remains the most serious problem facing western cardiology. In the USA alone, this cause of death removes 300 000 people from the population annually. It is presumed that the underlying cause is ventricular tachycardia or ventricular fibrillation, and so left ventricular function is perhaps the most important influence. However, the predictive value of left ventricular function, together with ambulatory ECG, is limited. Measures of autonomic function – heart rate variability and baroreflex sensitivity – may offer more hopeful possibilities. Increased sympathetic activity is damaging and interventions to modify autonomic activity may be a valuable means to limit the burden of sudden cardiac death.[37]

☐ Gene therapy

So much hyperbole has been written about gene transfer to the vascular system that I will refrain from adding more. However, Feldman and Isner provide a superb overview of the various approaches to gene treatment.[38]

Clearly, keeping abreast of developments in the basic science of cardioprotection is difficult if not impossible for cardiologists, let alone general clinicians. Detailed reviews published by *Science*[39] and *The Lancet*[40] provide helpful summaries of recent developments and future prospects.

■ CONCLUDING IN CONTEXT

The benefits achieved through drug therapy and other interventions, together with the exciting prospects of genetic and metabolic manipulations, should not obscure the gains from two other very simple behavioural changes: stopping smoking and increasing exercise.

In a provocative analysis of the benefits to be gained by risk factor intervention, Yudkin has shown that stopping smoking in men will reduce their 10-year mortality from coronary heart disease (currently at around 14.4 per 1000) by 2.74 per 1000.[41] The corresponding figures for antihypertensive treatment, cholesterol lowering and taking aspirin were 0.58, 0.82 and 2.64, respectively.

These gains are even larger among men with diabetes (20.84 per 1000 for those stopping smoking). Yudkin calculated that between 2400 and 3800 man-years of drug treatment would be required to prevent one death from CAD in a non-diabetic man. Rates of morbidity from progression to angina or non-fatal MI were not taken into account. Such a startling statistic as this should obscure neither the fact that drug treatment does save lives nor the importance of both the combined benefit of multiple risk factor intervention and targeting particular at-risk groups. Nevertheless, the doctor should be aware of the quantitative benefits of such a simple behavioural modification.

In terms of our pentagon of protection, exercise has the capacity to reduce both systolic and diastolic blood pressure,[42] increase HDL and reduce LDL plasma concentrations,[43] and diminish the risk of thromboembolic complications.[44] Lack of exercise may be quantitatively as important as smoking, hypertension and hypercholesterolaemia.[45]

Overall lifestyle is important in all aspects of intervention. For instance, the Treatment of Mild Hypertension Study (TOMHS)[46] showed that patients who lose weight, become more active, drink less alcohol and eat less salt had substantial reductions in blood pressure on drug treatment (mean reduction of 16 mmHg in systolic blood pressure and 12 mmHg in diastolic pressure). Drug treatment *combined* with lifestyle alterations is a highly effective therapeutic regimen. Stress is also implicated in hypertension[47] and atherosclerosis[48] in laboratory animals, and should be sought by the wise clinician who wishes to offer a complete programme of cardioprotective care.

The potential to reduce risk further has been measured in the UK in the ASPIRE study – Action on Secondary Prevention through Intervention to Reduce Events.[49] The design of ASPIRE involved a cross-sectional survey of coronary patients from a retrospective review of hospital records. Over 2500 patients were studied from four diagnostic categories – namely, coronary artery bypass grafting; PTCA; acute MI; and acute myocardial ischaemia without evidence of infarction. Risk factors and management details were noted from medical records; the control of risk factors was assessed at a patient interview 6 months after the event. The results were startling.

At interview, up to 37 per cent of patients were still smoking, three-quarters were overweight, up to 25 per cent were hypertensive, and over three-quarters had a total cholesterol above 5.2 mmol/l. Those individuals receiving treatment for blood glucose, cholesterol, and blood pressure had risk factor profiles little different from those not on treatment. Only one patient in three was taking a beta-blocker post-MI, and up to 20 per cent with ischaemia were not taking aspirin. The ASPIRE steering group concluded:

'There is considerable potential to reduce the risk of a further major ischaemic event in patients with established coronary disease. This can be achieved by effective lifestyle intervention, the rigorous management of blood pressure and cholesterol, and the appropriate use of prophylactic drugs.'

What better manifesto could there be for adopting a directly cardioprotective approach to patient management?

Our approach to cardioprotective therapeutics has focused on drugs, but occupational and social factors all operate to influence the atherosclerotic disease process. We hope that our integrated vision of cardioprotection will overcome the boundaries created by different specialties and emerging fashions. We continue to take an optimistic view of the future.

References

1. Kubler W, Haass M, Cardioprotection: definition, classification, and fundamental principles, *Heart* (1996) **75**:330–3.

2. Cohn JN, Archibald DG, Phil M et al, Effect of vasodilator therapy on mortality in chronic congestive heart failure – results of a Veterans Administration Cooperative Study, *N Engl J Med* (1986) **314**:1547–52.

3. Cohn J, Johnson G, Ziesche S et al, A comparison of enalapril with hydralazine–isosorbide dinitrate in the treatment of chronic congestive heart failure, *N Engl J Med* (1991) **325**:303–10.

4. Australia/New Zealand Heart Failure Research Collaborative Group, Randomised, placebo-controlled trial of carvedilol in patients with congestive heart failure due to ischaemic heart disease, *Lancet* (1997) **349**:375–80.

5. Packer M, Bristow M, Cohn J et al, The effect of carvedilol on morbidity and mortality in patients with chronic heart failure, *N Engl J Med* (1996) **334**:1349–55.

6. Hampton JR, van Veldhuisen DJ, Kleber FX et al, Randomised study of effect of ibopamine on survival in patients with advanced severe heart failure, *Lancet* (1997) **349**:971–77.

7. Niebauer J, Coats AJS, Treating chronic heart failure: time to take stock, *Lancet* (1997) **349**:966–7.

8. Doral HC, Nul DR, Grancelli HO et al, Randomised trial of low-dose amiodarone in severe congestive heart failure, *Lancet* (1994) **344**:493–8.

9. Singh SN, Fletcher RD, Fisher SG et al, Amiodarone in patients with congestive heart failure and asymptomatic ventricular fibrillation, *N Engl J Med* (1995) **333**:77–82.

10. Julian DG, Camm AJ, Frangin G et al, Randomised trial of effect of amiodarone on mortality in patients with left ventricular dysfunction after recent myocardial infarction: EMIAT, *Lancet* (1997) **349**:667–74.

11. Cairns JA, Connolly SJ, Roberts R et al, Randomised trial of outcome after myocardial infarction in patients with frequent or repetitive ventricular premature depolarisations: CAMIAT, *Lancet* (1997) **349**:675–82.

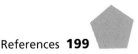

12. Pitt B, Segal R, Martinez FA et al, Randomised trial of losartan versus captopril in patients over 65 with heart failure (Evaluation of Losartan in the Elderly Study, ELITE), *Lancet* (1997) **349**:747–52.

13. Digitalis Investigation Group, The effect of digoxin on mortality and morbidity in patients with heart failure, *N Engl J Med* (1997) **336**:525–33.

14. Packer M, End of the oldest controversy in medicine: are we ready to conclude the debate on digitalis? *N Engl J Med* (1997) **336**:575–6.

15. Borhani NO, Mercuri M, Borhani PA et al, Final outcome results of the Multicenter Isradipine Diuretic Atherosclerosis Study (MIDAS), *JAMA* (1996) **276**:785–91.

16. Packer M, O'Connor CM, Ghali JK et al, Effect of amlodipine on morbidity and mortality in severe chronic heart failure, *N Engl J Med* (1996) **335**:1107–14.

17. The DEFIANT II Research Group, Doppler flow and echocardiography in functional cardiac insufficiency: assessment of nisoldipine therapy, *Eur Heart J* (1997) **18**:31–40.

18. Rengo F, Carbonin P, Pahor M et al, A controlled trial of verapamil in patients after acute myocardial infarction: results of the calcium antagonist reinfarction Italian study (CRIS), *Am J Cardiol* (1996) **77**:365–9.

19. Gong L, Zhang W, Zhu Y et al, Shanghai trial of nifedipine in the elderly (STONE), *J Hypertens* (1996) **14**:1237–45.

20. The HOT study group, The hypertension optimal treatment study (The HOT Study), *Blood Pressure* (1993) **2**:62–8.

21. Staessen JA, Fagard R, Thisj L et al, Randomized double blind comparison of placebo and active treatment for older patients with isolated systolic hypertension, *Lancet* (1997) **350**:757–64.

22. Kennedy HL, Rosenson RS, Physician use of beta-adrenergic blocking therapy: a changing perspective, *JACC* (1995) **26**:547–52.

23. Simoons ML, Deckers JW, New directions in anticoagulant and antiplatelet treatment, *Br Heart J* (1995) **74**:337–40.

24. The CAPTURE Investigators, Randomised placebo-controlled trial of abciximab before and during coronary intervention in refractory unstable angina: the CAPTURE study, *Lancet* (1997) **349**:1429–35.

25. CAPRIE Steering Committee, A randomized, blinded, trial of clopidogrel versus aspirin in patients at risk of ischaemic events (CAPRIE), *Lancet* (1996) **348**:1329–39.

26. Horton R, Cardiac stents: the next generation, *Lancet* (1996) **348**:601.

27. Fischman DL, Leon MB, Baim DS et al, A randomized comparison of coronary stent placement and balloon angioplasty in the treatment of coronary artery disease, *N Engl J Med* (1994) **331**:496–501.

28. Serruys PW, de Jaegere P, Kiemeneij F et al, A comparison of balloon-expandable stent implantation with balloon angioplasty in patients with coronary artery disease, *N Engl J Med* (1994) **331**:489–95.

28. Neumann FJ, Walter H, Richardt G, Schmitt C, Schomig A, Coronary Palmaz–Schatz stent implantation in acute myocardial infarction, *Heart* (1996) **75**:121–6.

30. The IMPACT-II investigators. Randomized placebo-controlled trial of effect of entifibatide on complications of percutaneous coronary intervention: IMPACT II, *Lancet* (1997) **349**:1422–28.

31. McCarthy M, Higher death rate found with aggressive treatment of non-Q-wave MIs, *Lancet* (1997) **349**:927.

32. Howard G, O'Leary DH, Zaccaro D et al, Insulin sensitivity and atherosclerosis, *Circulation* (1996) **93**:1809–17.

33. Reaven GM, Chen Y-DI, Insulin resistance, its consequences, and coronary heart disease: must we choose one culprit? *Circulation* (1996) **93**:1780–3.

34. Mayer EL, Jacobsen DW, Robinson K, Homocysteine and coronary atherosclerosis, *JACC* (1996) **27**:517–27.

35. Przyklenk K, Kloner RA, Preconditioning: a balanced perspective, *Br Heart J* (1995) **74**:575–7.

36. Bhagat K, Vallance P, Invariable nitric oxide synthase in the cardiovascular system, *Heart* (1996) **75**:218–20.

37. Barron HV, Lesh MD, Autonomic nervous system and sudden cardiac death, *JACC* (1996) **27**:1053–60.

38. Feldman LJ, Isner JM, Gene therapy for the vulnerable plaque, *JACC* (1995) **26**:826–35.

39. Cardiovascular medicine, *Science* (1996) **272**:663–93.

40. Coronary heart disease, *Lancet* (1996) **348** (suppl I): 1–31.

41. Yudkin JS, How can we best prolong life? Benefits of coronary risk factor reduction in non-diabetic and diabetic subjects, *Br Med J* (1993) **306**:1313–18.

42. Nelson L, Jennings GL, Ecler MD, Komer PI, Effect of changing levels of physical inactivity on blood pressure and haemodynamics in essential hypertension, *Lancet* (1986) **ii**:473–6.

43. Hardman AE, Hudson J, Jones PRM, Norgan NG, Brisk walking and high density lipoprotein cholesterol concentration in formerly sedentary women, *Br Med J* (1989) **299**:1204–5.

44. Ferguson EW, Bernier LL, Barton GR, Yu-Yehiro J, Schoomaker EB, Effects of exercise and conditioning on clotting and fibrinolytic activity in men, *J Appl Physiol* (1987) **62**:1416–21.

45. Powell KE, Thompson DD, Casperson CJ, Kendrick JS, Physical activity and the incidence of coronary heart disease, *Ann Rev Public Health* (1987) **8**:253–87.

46. Goldsmith MF, Treatment of mild hypertension study shows results better when drugs abet lifestyle changes, *JAMA* (1993) **269**:323–4.

47. Henry JP, Ely DL, Stephens PM et al, The role of psychosocial factors in the development of arteriosclerosis in CBA mice, *Atherosclerosis* (1971) **14**:203–6.

48. Kaplan JR, Manuck SB, Clarkson TB, Lusso FM, Tarb DM, Social status, environment, and atherosclerosis in cynomolgus monkeys, *Arteriosclerosis* (1982) **2**:359–64.

49. ASPIRE Steering Group, A British Cardiac Society survey of the potential for the secondary prevention of coronary disease: ASPIRE (Action on Secondary Prevention through Intervention to Reduce Events), Principal results, *Heart* (1996) **75**:334–42.

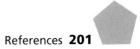

Index

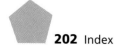

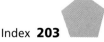

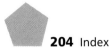

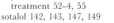

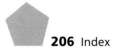